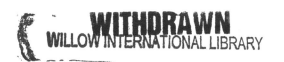

No Family History

New Social Formations
Series Editor:
Charles Lemert, Wesleyan University

No Family History

The Environmental Links to Breast Cancer

Sabrina McCormick

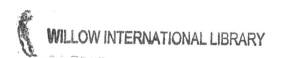

WILLOW INTERNATIONAL LIBRARY

ROWMAN & LITTLEFIELD PUBLISHERS, INC.
Lanham • Boulder • New York • Toronto • Plymouth, UK

For my Dad who taught me to stand up and fight

For my Mom who taught me what to fight for

ROWMAN & LITTLEFIELD PUBLISHERS, INC.

Published in the United States of America
by Rowman & Littlefield Publishers, Inc.
A wholly owned subsidiary of The Rowman & Littlefield Publishing Group, Inc.
4501 Forbes Boulevard, Suite 200, Lanham, Maryland 20706
www.rowmanlittlefield.com

Estover Road
Plymouth PL6 7PY
United Kingdom

British Library Cataloguing in Publication Information Available

Library of Congress Cataloging-in-Publication Data:

McCormick, Sabrina.
 No family history : the environmental links to breast cancer / Sabrina McCormick.
  p. ; cm. — (New social formations)
 Includes bibliographical references and index.
 ISBN 978-0-7425-6408-4 (cloth : alk. paper)
 ISBN 978-0-7425-6628-6 (electronic)
 1. Breast—Cancer—Environmental aspects. I. Title. II. Series.
 [DNLM: 1. Breast Neoplasms—etiology—United States. 2. Environmental
Exposure—adverse effects—United States. 3. Breast Neoplasms—prevention &
control—United States. 4. Public Policy—United States. WP 870 M4775n 2009]
 RC280.B8M3556 2009
 616.99'449071—dc22   2008050133

Printed in the United States of America

∞™ The paper used in this publication meets the minimum requirements of American
National Standard for Information Sciences—Permanence of Paper for Printed Library
Materials, ANSI/NISO Z39.48-1992.

Contents

Introduction

When I was eight, I lost everything—and almost my mother too. My room and all the stuff in it—toys, dance costumes, purple barrettes, green tights, sparkly lip gloss—I had to leave behind when we abandoned our house on Bishop Lake. The cornflower blue cottage was perched on a leaf-strewn hill at the edge of a narrow gravel road. My room with its grass-green carpet and rainbow wall mural sat at the bottom of the hill under the living room. Its windows looked out over foggy green water that was fresh and inviting on hot days. The placid lake in suburban Marietta, Georgia, had formerly been a vacation colony for the rich, recently adopted by the middle class for year-round use.

I could see my friend Dru's house across the water. She had a tire swing. On balmy days we would fly through the air and drop into the warm water, in love with summer vacation. Cooler days had us scouting nature's most exciting jewels—mice, grasshoppers, and spindly lizards. I spent the first half of the summer of 1983 at my father's home in a neighboring town. In July, I returned to the lake. It did not welcome me back. My mother was sick. She could not feel her hands. Her lips tingled. She felt dizzy. Then one night a few months later, she let us know something was wrong. We had to move away from the Bishop Lake house immediately, leaving everything behind. I imagined our home being preserved like the Gardner Museum, Edison's home, or any celebrity's dwelling for generations to see and not touch. In fact, our belongings were to be disposed of as toxic waste, dumped in a landfill, preserved in a coffin of garbage.

My ten-year-old brother and I did not understand. We were still traumatized by our parents' divorce three years earlier. At that time I had taken all of my choice toys to Mom's. Now they were gone. While I was with my father, a crew had sprayed our cottage beams for powder post beetles. It seemed innocent enough. My mom left while the crew worked. Afterward she let the house air out, and everything should have been fine. But the crew had illegally used a cancerous chemical, chlordane.

Believing the crew's claims that they had sprayed a safe chemical, my mother dragged the soaked plastic sheets covering the carpet outdoors and wiped dripping chemical residue from the walls. Her symptoms appeared almost immediately, but she ignored them. A tart odor soaked the air for weeks. Worried about the stench and her worsening symptoms, my mother had a chunk of beam tested. The report showed high levels of chlordane. That night we moved into a hotel.

Before 1983, 3.6 million pounds of chlordane were applied to corn, fruits, lawns, and houses every year. It was used to exterminate termites and beetles. But the initial testing of chlordane, like that of many other chemicals, was not sufficient. Eventually, the Environmental Protection Agency began examining air, drinking water, and soil all of which contained and continue to be contaminated by the chemical. By 1983, the agency had found that it caused damage to the nervous and blood systems, lungs, and kidney and that it might cause leukemia and cancer. That year, regulations were put in place to ban chlordane.

Chlordane is one chemical included in the list of substances proven to cause cancer. Scientists do not know how much of these chemicals humans have to encounter to get sick or how much you have to inhale or absorb through your skin by touching them on contaminated surfaces. My mother did not know either. She just knew that her children were at risk and that we should not be exposed.

I forgot about chlordane and stopped thinking about Bishop Lake as I got older. The fear of getting sick, the childlike sense of extreme loss, grew dim as I moved on to more important things, like learning to drive, making my parents crazy, and going to college. By my mid-twenties, those memories were distant and unformed, a vague halo of consciousness in my mind that was becoming more focused on the future and a career choice.

Soon after my twenty-fifth birthday, I began a doctorate in sociology at Brown University, not entirely sure of what I would do with the degree but simply knowing that I liked to ask questions and was driven by a deeply ingrained sense of social justice. I first worked with Phil Brown, a professor who had just begun research on how some diseases were beginning to be regarded as environmentally caused. One of them was breast cancer. As I researched background on the disease, I realized that ending up at Brown was not a coincidence. My childhood loss had shaped how the rest of my life would play out.

Studies of our rodent friends show that chlordane is one of many chemicals that cause breast cancer (Mills and Yang 2005). My young age at exposure made things worse, as my still-developing body was more vulnerable then than now. A great deal of evidence shows that being exposed to these substances at a young age, in particular, increases the risk of getting disease (Jenkins et al. 2007; Kajekar 2007). Many other women, even without the experience I had as a child, fit a similar bill. In fact, all of us have been exposed to carcinogenic chemicals to a greater or lesser degree. These substances are ubiquitous—in cleaning products, piping that circulates water in cities, cosmetics—you name it (Harvey and Darbre 2004; Markey et al. 2002). They encompass our lives, our every breath. The science proving a link between many of these chemicals and breast cancer is hotly debated. While some scientists hold that enough research has been done, others argue that there is a solid body of evidence on which new regulations should be based.

These debates mask a political economy of disease—a vast, powerful group of corporations protected by weak governmental practices that have shaped what we are exposed to every day. What we know and what we take seriously have been intimately shaped by this political economy. A rising tide of activists has argued that contemporary trends in research have left us in the dark. Political economy of disease is not an abstraction. It affects everyday lives and deaths.

A SCIENTIFIC AND POLITICAL ECONOMY OF BREAST CANCER

In this book, I argue that a vast political economy of disease has caused us to focus on treatment, detection, and cure while missing a more difficult and political piece of the puzzle—how to *prevent* breast cancer. While many other books have shown the experience of breast cancer or the available treatments, this book is different in that it shows how politics and money shape responses to disease. Political economy refers to the interrelationship between industry, our market-based economic system, and political institutions. These institutions often prioritize major corporate interests instead of the public's health and well-being. So the political economy of disease highlights the links between political institutions and a capitalist system (Caporaso and Levine 1992).

Since the emergence of a capitalist economy, there has always been a political economy in America where there are interconnections between corporations and government institutions. Health policy and scientific endeavors are two pieces of this puzzle. The "war on cancer" is also embedded in it.

President Nixon began the "war" in 1971 (Sporn 1996). Scientists are little closer to finding a cure for breast cancer now than they were back then. Many realize that and feel as hopeless as the daughter watching her mother waste away in the last moments of stage 4 breast cancer. While treatment is critical to addressing the thousands of cases of breast cancer that emerge every year, the quest for effective drugs is driven not only by sympathy but also by economics. There is a great deal of money to be made from treatment, while few people see profit in prevention. As a result, certain kinds of information about the disease have proliferated. Mostly, it tells *individual* women what to do to prevent the illness (Brown et al. 2001) or offers them treatments they can take once they get the disease. The massive costs to patients are actually profits for their producers. Unfortunately, most of these treatments have partially beneficial results at best (Bonadonna et al. 1995; Goldhirsch et al. 2001).

All this information about individual responsibility for prevention and treatment is marketed by a powerful public relations industry that coats the profit motive with pink—pink ribbons, pink shoes, pink teddy bears, and endless other pink products. These marketers do an excellent job of disguising how the very same corporations that make cures or raise funds for research also produce carcinogenic products (Houlihan et al. 2002). This profit circle is so masked that it is hard to tell where the money comes from and where it really goes (Clorfene-Casten 1996). By focusing on fund-raising and treatment and pushing for more and more research, these large-scale industries put pressure on women to prevent their own cancer rather than recognizing the need for corporate accountability and corporate culpability. Their well-funded campaigns distract walkers, runners, shoppers, and victims from looking at what might have caused cancer in the first place—exposures in the environment. We change our diets. We exercise. We get mammograms. We also walk, shop, and race for a cure. We know what pink stands for. It means breast cancer. It means raising money. It means finding a cure. The fact is that we are missing the boat.

The political economy of breast cancer includes those who are making money from breast cancer and their problematic influence over the political institutions meant to protect us from it. For example, drug companies that develop and manufacture medicine for prevention or treatment of breast cancer represent a multi-billion-dollar industry. AstraZeneca, manufacturer of some of the most popular breast cancer drugs, has an annual revenue of around $19 billion. In 2004, the company made $519 million through sales of just a single breast cancer drug, Arimidex (AstraZeneca 2004), a drug that lowers the amount of estrogen in the body, therefore possibly decreasing breast cancer risk. Through a well-organized lobbying program, financial support, and its easy passage through Food and Drug Administration channels, AstraZeneca has direct relationships with the state and many nonprofits, influencing policies and how nonprofit education campaigns are conducted (Batt and Gross 1999).

The idea of a political economy may seem abstract and distant, a theory that has little impact on our own realities. But we are all subject to it. When a scientist pursues funding for breast cancer research and finds support available only for treatment, she is responding to the political economy of disease. When we are forced to buy vegetables sprayed with carcinogenic pesticides, we are subjected to political economy. Symbols transmit the political economy on a more intimate, personal level. They have even been developed to represent certain ways of thinking about the disease (Kolker 2004). These symbols encompass our lives and embed themselves in our consciousness. The pink ribbon, with its implication of hope and cure is the most ubiquitous and emotionally poignant. Social interactions between friends and family members, doctors and patients, and consumers and sellers of pink products are bound to these symbols. When a daughter responds to emotional distress about her mother getting breast cancer by attending a walk for a cure rather than writing a letter to her congressman demanding investigation of causes, she is reacting to the options provided by these institutions and represented in symbols.

Recently, scholars have argued that an analysis of political economy is too limited and that technology and science represent greater power in our society than just dollars (Castells 1997; Knorr-Cetina 1999). Especially in the case of illnesses, where science and technology are looked to as the source of progress and healing, political economy may seem less important. However, these two concepts are not contradictory. I argue that political economy, science, and technology overlap and intersect, resulting in a "scientific economy," or a set of research findings and technological tools that directly benefit large financial and political interests. One way this works is when state-funded studies evaluate the efficacy of treatments, and corporations use that knowledge to develop more lucrative products (Angell 2004). In the meantime, the lab tools used to reach these conclusions get refined to make traditional science profitable for corporations (Brown et al. 2006). The "scientific economy" of breast cancer has resulted in a focus on profitable detection and treatment strategies rather than assessing how we might prevent the disease. In the case of breast cancer and many other illnesses, these factors—politics, money and science—mean that rates will rise while people will stay alive only through the grueling experience of treatments.

Breaking these trends and developing new institutions that might prevent rather than only treat disease is difficult because of cultural, scientific, economic, and political constraints. However, in the case of breast cancer, this is being done (McCormick et al. 2003). Brave individuals have led this movement. They have spoken out about the causes of the growing breast cancer epidemic. Rachel Carson (1961) said,

> Today we find our world filled with cancer-producing agents. An attack on cancer that is concentrated wholly or even largely on therapeutic measures . . . will fail because it leaves untouched the great reservoirs of carcinogenic agents which would continue to claim new victims. (241)

The famous poet Audre Lorde (1980) wrote from her hospital bed,

> Cancer is not just another degenerative and unavoidable disease of the ageing process. It has distinct and identifiable causes, and these are mainly exposures to chemicals or physical agents in the environment. (73)

Scientist and writer Sandra Steingraber (1998) wrote,

> Banned pesticides, like fugitives from justice, have not entirely disappeared. We have forgotten about them, but they are still among us. They frequent foreign ports. They languish underground. But they are beginning to surface again in the tissues of women with breast cancer. (10)

Sentinels to the new fight over breast cancer, these women are reshaping the debate about breast cancer—rather than arguing about which lifestyle factor is best or when to start mammography, they question what the causes are. Scientists, public officials, and women with breast cancer have begun to devote attention to the environmental *causes* of disease in order to generate a new understanding of how to respond to the epidemic. The second section of this book tells their stories and what they have been able to achieve. They have drawn attention to why breast cancer rates are skyrocketing by paying attention to environmental causes. Researchers are developing new scientific tools and methods in order to detect exposures never previously considered but common to most women's lives (Rudel et al. 2007).

While the vast majority of research funding, awareness campaigns, and political campaigns take the traditional approach focused on detection, treatment, and cure (Brown et al. 2006; Gardner 2006), this new set of researchers, advocates, and political leaders have turned to issues of prevention (McCormick et al. 2003). These women and men are investigating what in the air, food, and water could be the culprits. Their findings often fly in the face of traditional explanations of why so many women die every year.

These pioneering individuals, research institutes, and organizations represent the little voice of breast cancer. Even the prestigious names Harvard, Stanford, and Columbia do not guarantee them fame or media attention. Although activists have supported these innovative scientific ventures, compared to those researching pharmaceuticals or detection, the funding they receive is a pittance (Breast Cancer Fund 2000). The number of protective policies these scientists and activists have pushed forward is, in relative terms, minute. Their organizations are often struggling. Bucking trends in research, risking their credibility, and running the race for tenure, they have tracked down meager funds to look for a cause. Yet despite their findings that reach across diverse scientific fields, many think the causes of breast cancer are unknown. This is not the case.

The third section of this book connects breast cancer to the broader landscape of illnesses in the United States. In it, I explain why the politics of breast cancer also have important ramifications for many other illnesses. Prostate, uterine, and other reproductive cancers as well as developmental disorders are linked to the same substances that have led to the rise in breast cancer over the years (Birnbaum and Fenton 2003). Many of these other cancers are skyrocketing upward.

The answers for decreasing breast cancer rates are the same for all these diseases. The answers are both simple and complex. Simply put, these chemicals should be used less and regulated more. State governments and the European Union are already pursuing tougher regulatory standards despite the counterefforts of a powerful chemical and industrial lobby (Pearce and Tombs 1996; Reuters 2002). However, finding alternatives may be complicated. Many of these chemicals are fundamental to industrial production, so safer alternatives must be developed. Innovations are in progress through fields like green chemistry, but significant government investment will be necessary to bring these new, safer products to market. Possibilities for making our world less toxic and safer abound. It is simply a matter of investing in our own futures.

I

SECTION I

Chapter One

What We Do about Breast Cancer

Robin looked into the mirror on the medicine cabinet, but it was too high. She could see the shadow cast under her armpit but nothing lower. She raised her arm and leaned back against the wall. The light switch jabbed mercilessly into her shoulder blade. She could still not see her breast. She could feel the lump but could not see it.

It was starting to get dark outside. The last light shot through slivers of sea grass shifting and swaying along the edge of the cul-de-sac. Shrill children's voices pierced the soft brushing sound of the grasses. Robin could see little Eddy and Tori, the two youngest, pushing their go-carts out of the street and into the driveway. Brittany was already inside, trudging up the stairs to her room, a backpack thumping against each stair behind her. Robin pulled her turquoise green tank top back over her left breast and checked in the small, square mirror one last time.

She still looked young, with her cheeks only beginning to ripple when she smiled. At this time of year, her skin was pale. The spring wind had been too crisp to take one of Eddy's boats out on the sound, and she had not had time to sit by herself next to their backyard swimming pool. Even without the sun, white highlights already streaked Robin's thick yellow blond mane. The hairdresser figured that summer would arrive soon, and Robin had given her free reign. Not long ago it had been a burnt red, closer to her real hair color.

Like her face, her body was still youthful, although keeping it up meant being on the Stairmaster and lifting weights for a few hours most days during the week. Robin's breasts, one of the few body parts that couldn't be improved at the gym, seemed like they had not faced three hungry mouths. Implants had helped with that. They were more than ten years old. The operation had made her breasts firm and lusciously taut, giving new life to what had then been twenty-nine-year-old flesh. An arch sloped gracefully down the front of her body from a sharp collarbone without a single wrinkle. At forty-three, Robin knew they were beautiful, although after having children she cared less.

There had never been any problems with the implants, and the doctors were telling her now that the bump she could feel was nothing to worry about, that it was just something women get. But it kept bothering her. Like an underwire bra whose metal lacing had escaped its cage, the lump poked through her chest, grazing her arm. It was annoying, if nothing else. She wanted to take it out, make it go away.

Breast cancer did not cross her mind. The thing just needed to be gotten rid of.

I had met Robin only a few weeks before, five years after beginning graduate school. We met when I decided to make a documentary film that portrayed my research. A breast cancer activist on Long Island, Lorraine Pace, had connected me with Robin. Lorraine is one of the loudest women with breast cancer on the island. Her sonorous voice and demanding nature have helped bring attention to women's concerns about high rates on the peninsula. She knows everyone in the area, even if they don't always like her. The film needed a character in Long Island who could show viewers the real experience of breast cancer, so I called Lorraine to ask if she knew anyone undergoing treatment. She called back within an hour. I will never forget what she said.

"I know four women who were diagnosed this week," Lorraine left on my voice mail. "They all live pretty close to me. I will check if any of them will talk to you and call you back." I had been back and forth to Long Island from Rhode Island for several years, knew activists in many parts of the island, and had heard their stories of getting breast cancer, having a recurrence, and fighting it again. But this was my introduction to the reality of the disease. Constant diagnoses. No explanation of why. This was one of the reasons I was in graduate school: to find out what was causing so much breast cancer and why no one seemed to be doing anything about it.

THE BREAST CANCER IMPERATIVE

Today in the United States, a woman is diagnosed with breast cancer every three minutes. Another woman will die every eleven minutes (Evans 2006). The epidemic has been rising for the past sixty years (DeBruin and Josephy 2002). Not slowly but rapidly, breast cancer has taken an increasing number of women's lives—not only the old and frail but also the young and healthy, mothers with small children, and leaders in every field. In 1940, around one in twenty-four women who lived to be eighty was afflicted. In 1964, one in twenty women who lived to be age eighty would get the disease (Evans 2006). By 2006, that number reached one in eight. Breast cancer is the most common killer of middle-aged women in the United States, Canada, and northern Europe. There were an estimated 184,450 cases of invasive breast cancer diagnosed in 2008 alone (American Cancer Society [ACS] 2008) (see table 1.1). Almost all breast cancer cases are in women. Only 1 percent strike men (ACS 2006a). So familiar is breast cancer in American culture that television shows, public figures, and popular culture reflect its existence. In 1997, Murphy Brown was diagnosed with the disease, maybe one of the first fictional accounts. More recently, Samantha, the sexy dynamo in the popular *Sex in the City*, suffered the same fate in the show's last season. Awareness has proliferated, yet the number of lives lost adds up year after year.

As a society, we face a mandate to heal the many women and men who get sick each year. This chapter begins to introduce how breast cancer is dealt with, including our major medical and societal responses to it, why we have chosen them, and how they are often shortsighted. First, I briefly explain what breast cancer is and who it impacts. I then describe, again in brief, the detection and treatment regimens common today. By taking a step back to look at this work from afar, we can see the fault lines in medical advice and preventive treatment regimens. Advice is driven by a medical paradigm focused on lifestyle and detached from other risk factors outside of an individual's day-to-day actions. This leaves certain other considerations generally ignored—in

Table 1.1.   Number of Breast Cancer Cases (for Women), 1940–2004

Year	Total Number of New Cases	New in situ Cases	Estimated Number of Deaths
2004	215,990	59,390	40,110
2003	211,300	55,700	39,800
2002	203,500	54,300	39,600
2001	192,200	47,100	40,200
2000	182,800	Not reported	40,800
1999	175,000	39,900	43,300
1998	178,700	36,900	43,500
1980	187,000	*	*
1940	69,000	*	*

Note: This data was partially gathered from the American Cancer Society.
* No data available.

particular, those that center around environmental causes in the shape of chemicals and exposures in everyday life. This chapter lays the groundwork for the rest of the book. It helps explain how we handle breast cancer today so that we can think about what new directions might be approached.

The one term used for breast cancer actually refers to a family of different diseases (Mayo Clinic 2005). There are different types of cell growth, like estrogen positive or estrogen negative, and various sites in the breast where these new, unhealthy cells rear their ugly heads, like the duct or the gland. What they all have in common is uncontrollable cancerous cell growth in the breast. Like other cancers, this growth can move out of the area of the breast into any other part of the body in a form of metastases. Publicized breast cancer rates generally do not include a particular type of cases—those that are in situ. These are called a precursor to cancerous growth and therefore not added to total numbers. However, in situ cases have been climbing even more rapidly than invasive cancers (Devra Davis, personal communication, 2007).

The majority of work around breast cancer goes into improving detection and treatment and to finding a cure. Mammography is the most common form of detection (Rakowski and Clark 1998). Treatments range from surgical interventions like mastectomy and lumpectomy to radiation and chemotherapy. All these methods of detection and treatment have extended women's lives and been celebrated as important advances. However, calling this progress has been hotly debated because, while treatments extend lives, the cost is high. This rhetoric of progress disguises the real toll such treatments have on women and their families.

DETECTING BREAST CANCER

"Detection is your best protection" is a quote frequently used by breast cancer organizations and medical advisers. Promotion of mammography is the most predominant public message. Mammography is consequently growing in use. Demand is so great that it has become a profession in itself. Reed Dunnick, chair of the Department of Radiology at the University of Michigan, explains that "1,000 new radiologists are trained each year" (Dunnick 2005). Facilities have also grown. In 2003, there were 8,600 mammography facilities in the United States (National Academy of Sciences 2003). A massive number of machines have been manufactured to serve the populations demanding the exam. They are not cheap. Each digital mammography machine costs around $350,000. Analog machines range from $75,000 to $100,000 (May et al. 2001). An exam costs $100, in many states paid in tax dollars. Massive investments have been made in making mammography the thrust of protection against breast cancer. The costs to women who need the exam or the government subsidizing it are not low. In total, mammography usage is estimated to cost $5 billion to $13 billion per year (Ransom 2006). These monies go to companies that manufacture machines, technicians who provide the service, and hospitals that offer space where exams are conducted.

Proponents claim that getting a mammogram can save your life. However, this is greatly debated. While data show that getting a mammogram extends women's lives, other studies show that is not true. In 2001, Joyce C. Lashof, chair of a committee reporting on mammography from the National Academy of Sciences Institute of Medicine, announced that it could reduce cancer deaths by 30 percent at most (Institute of Medicine 2001). Many argue that since the 1960s, when it was first touted by the government, the exam has become better regulated and technicians have become more qualified (Pisano et al. 2000). However, as the National Institute of Medicine explained in its 2001 report, the number of deaths prevented has not changed since the initial landmark study of mammography usage forty years ago. Mammograms miss 10 to 25 percent of tumors (Destounis et al. 2004; Kopans 1992). This is because some breast cancers do not show up on mammograms; rather, they "hide" in dense breast tissue (Qaseem et al. 2007). A normal (or negative) study is not a guarantee that a woman is cancer free. The false-negative rate is estimated to be 15 to 20 percent, higher in younger women and women with dense breasts (Kerlikowske 1996). Most research has shown that mammograms catch cancer faster than a breast self-exam (Hackshaw and Paul 2003), but, surprisingly, earlier detection does not necessarily mean better survival rates (Miller et al. 2000). It often does mean less aggressive treatments.

Another problem with mammography as a diagnostic tool is that some early cancers detected are completely benign (Epstein et al. 2001). For example, in situ cases are detected by mammography, but 75 percent of these cases do not become invasive (Hadjiiski et al. 2004). Those women undergo the mental stress and anguish of a diagnosis with no resultant disease. False-positive readings are also possible. In other words, breast biopsies may be recommended on the basis of a mammogram and find no cancer.

Mammography may actually increase breast cancer risk. The exam uses a low dose of radiation that is risky especially for younger women whose breast tissue is more vulnerable (Bradbury and Olopade 2006). Radiation is one of the well-substantiated causes of breast cancer (Doody et al. 2000). Even in 1978, the National Cancer Institute (NCI) informed women with breast cancer that "mammograms may also increase a woman's chances of breast cancer." Judith Shills (1988), the editor of the *FDA Drug Bulletin*, wrote, "Because the radiation from the mammography can itself cause increased risk of breast cancer, researchers are continually trying to develop ways to reduce the amount of radiation from the procedure." Over the years the exam has been in use, the amount of radiation emitted in any procedure has decreased. Shills wrote, "In the last several years, the average radiation exposure from mammography in the United States has been reduced about 50 percent." Promoters argue that this amount is minimal. However, the cumulative exposure over a lifetime can be great. If a woman begins having mammograms at age forty and lives to be age eighty, she has been exposed to an excess of radiation.

In this sense and others, the age at which women first start having mammograms plays an important role in the debate about whether to use mammograms for detection. While the Food and Drug Administration once recommended fifty as a start age, the ACS has now moved that to age forty (Qaseem et al. 2007). That age has dropped to forty and even thirty-five for women with a family history of the disease. The younger the woman, the more vulnerable her tissue is to the radiation, and the more likely the exposure will cause cancer (Aisenberg et al. 2000; Kelsey and Bernstein 1996). Scientists continue to debate the appropriate age, while the ACS and the NCI publicly promote the procedure for women age forty and up.

Despite these drawbacks to mammography, it is the most cost-effective method of detection available to doctors today. Although other technologies, like magnetic resonance imaging and sonograms, could be used to detect cancerous growths, the long history of using mammography makes it the currently predominant strategy. As Barron Lerner, professor of medicine and public health at Columbia University, recounts in *The Breast Cancer Wars* (2001), a broad-sweeping campaign by the ACS, backed up by manufacturers of mammography film and machines, instigated the widespread usage of mammography. Government agencies like the NCI, in conjunction with nonprofits like the ACS, began promoting the exam in the 1960s. The ACS began advertising mammography in 1982 (Stabiner 1997), and the government has subsidized its usage since 1990. A congressional act passed that year provided funding for women to be screened who did not otherwise have access and for disseminating clear messages about the importance of early detection. In the first year, 1992, there were 572 sites where women could be screened. The next year, there were 1,305—more than a 200 percent increase. As of January 1993, the Centers for Disease Control and Prevention had screened 31,105 women; 2,774 of those women were referred for follow-up, and 102 women were diagnosed (House of Representatives 1993). These numbers have grown massively over time. In 2005, 74.6 percent of women in America got a mammogram (Ryerson et al. 2007). More women are taking advantage of this resource, and there is less questioning of it.

FINDING THE LUMP

In April, three months before I met Robin, while I was celebrating my thirtieth birthday, she was experiencing the most frightening moment in her life. She had felt something in her chest and gone to have it tested. Her mammogram detected a lump. She was only forty-three, on the young side for a diagnosis of cancer. Her doctor assured her that it was nothing and told her to go home and have a good summer. She went home but did not forget about it. The lump jabbed her in the side. It felt wrong. She went back and demanded to know if it was cancerous. This meant a biopsy. She and Eddy went to the local hospital, and she was put under.

"I was sitting in the waiting room, watching television, and the phone rang. It was crazy the way the phone would ring and one of us would answer it, waiting to find out what happened." Eddy had waited while the doctors anesthetized Robin and took a tissue sample from her tumor. When she awoke from the surgery, the doctor had told her the same thing that he had said to Eddy over the heavy pink plastic phone in the waiting room.

"He said to me, 'Your wife has cancer'! Just like that!" Eddy's face turned red, remembering. "I said, 'You must have the wrong person,' and hung up."

That first surgery was followed by two other, more invasive attempts to remove the cancerous tumor in her left breast. Each time, the surgeons were unsure that all the cancerous cells had been cut away. Robin made a final decision. Only one more surgery. She would have both breasts removed. There would be no chance that cancer was left in her body.

It would be hard for the family. All the kids were school age but home for the summer. Eddy was gone during the day, and Robin kept everything going in the household. This would be impossible after having invasive surgery. Although they lived comfortably on Long Island, Eddy and Robin faced the same financial constraints as most young families wanting to give as much as possible to the kids but never having as much as they would like. There would be no paid help. No nurse, no child care, no help with the cleaning. The family would continue to depend on Robin.

TREATING BREAST CANCER

Like detecting breast cancer, treatment is a multi-billion-dollar industry (Ehrenreich 2001). The first and most historically predominant treatment was the Halstead radical mastectomy. Surgeons have been using this procedure for hundreds of years. Medical records reflect how grapefruit-size growths were cut away from women's breasts even before anesthesia was invented (Lerner 2001). By the time it was put to use, it meant emotional trauma for women with a suspicious lump. They were put under anesthesia with two breasts not knowing if, on waking, they would have either. In possibly the first step in breast cancer activism, Babette Rosomond made sure all women could choose for themselves.

Rosomond was possibly the Rosa Parks of breast cancer activism. Although she lacked the kind of organizational support provided by the burgeoning civil rights movement, like Rosa she refused to be told what to do. Prior to the biopsy of her potentially malignant breast tumor, rather than sign the release form allowing the surgeon to immediately perform a radical mastectomy, Babette requested that she be allowed to wait several days between the first and second procedures (Lerner 2001). Her surgeon argued against the delay, claiming that it would mean her life. This simple yet seemingly life-threatening action eventually resulted in informed consent laws mandating that patients be allowed to decline medical procedures or choose which one to have. Thanks to Babette, surgeons get a patient's permission.

As surgical practices improved, treatments became easier. By 1979, the radical mastectomy was replaced by the modified radical mastectomy, which meant the removal of less tissue under the arm and in the chest. It was a difficult transition for surgeons who felt that cancer cells might be missed if less tissue was removed. But this was not necessarily the case. Between 1958, when data were first collected about the efficacy of surgical procedures, and twenty years later, when modified mastectomies began, there was a burgeoning of scientific studies that dealt with this question. A growing amount of evidence showed that a radical mastectomy was unnecessarily invasive (Fisher 1970). But long before there was scientific consensus, individual researchers and women felt strongly that the radical mastectomy was an outmoded procedure. Many mastectomies performed from 1977 to 1979 could have been avoided. Medical transitions like this reflect how waiting for scientific consensus often causes pain for individuals whose lives are intimately connected to what that science dictates. A similar bumpy transition to the lumpectomy took place in the 1980s. In 1985, scientists concluded that the lumpectomy plus radiation was equivalent to mastectomy for breast cancer. This procedure began to become more and more widespread, so that today the lumpectomy is common practice. Awareness about choices pushed changes in surgical practices.

Today, surgery is combined with breast cancer drugs or can be avoided completely by pharmaceutical interventions that are the latest set of treatments. There is a range of such drugs, including those to reduce the risk of getting the disease, such as cyclophosphamide, or those to use during breast

cancer treatment, such as Zoladex. Others can be taken posttreatment to reduce the risk of a recurrence. These advances have been celebrated and
pointed to as the steps toward making breast cancer obsolete. Millions of dollars of funding go into making treatments like these and others less difficult.
But as Dr. Freya Schnabel, the director of Columbia University's Breast Cancer Center, says, "Breast cancer does not go away quickly. The treatments
sometimes go on for an extended period of time. The woman with the disease
as well as the family is highly affected." She has been treating these patients
for years, has seen every type of case, and knows what is most common. Advances in breast cancer treatment have extended lives. But the cost of what
many call the "breast cancer epidemic" is still high.

STRATEGIES FOR PREVENTION

Most publicity has been directed toward detection and treatment. Despite the
emotional, physical, and financial cost of breast cancer, there has been little
focus on primary prevention. Perhaps we are too busy taking care of the millions of women living with breast cancer today to take a different approach.
Maybe the upcoming hundreds of thousands of new cases that will occur next
year seem like enough to handle. As doctor and author Ronald Glasser (2004)
says, "Prevention comes secondary to just keeping people alive."

The idea of prevention is based on the goal of decreasing risk. According
to the ACS, one of the most prominent voices in public education, there are
several prominent lifestyle "choices" that women can make in order to decrease breast cancer risk (ACS 2006). The ACS says that being slightly overweight, having children after thirty, not exercising in youth, taking the birth
control pill, drinking, taking hormone replacement therapy, and not breast-
feeding are all lifestyle choices that increase breast cancer risk. The idea is
that decisions can be made to decrease these risks. While some of these preventive strategies are actually not clearly choices, others are preventive
strategies that act as a deterrent for many illnesses, such as eating well, exercising, staying thin, not smoking, and avoiding too much alcohol.

Despite how basic they may seem, these pieces of advice are debated. For
example, lowering fat consumption and losing weight are commonly given
on the list of things to do, like performing breast self-exams and getting mammograms. But this broad-sweeping advice may mask important complexities.
The reason for a possible link between fat and cancer is not understood. One
question raised by many breast cancer advocates is whether incalculably per-
vasive hormones in American beef, residing primarily in fat, are contributing
to cancer. American beef is so plagued by hormones that the European Union

pays millions of dollars to the United States in trade tariffs every year in or-der to keep it out of Europe (Mills 2002). American consumers are less aware of this scourge, and the Food and Drug Administration has allowed these chemicals to be pumped into the bloodstream of cattle and the American food market—meaning us. Although research is emerging that links these hor-mones to breast cancer (Hakinson et al. 1998), the public is largely in the dark. And for women, advice is rarely given about which fat to consume de-spite the fact that it's specifically fat from red meat that increases risk.

Recombinant bovine growth hormone (RBGH) is one very controversial chemical in American beef linked to breast cancer. It is injected into the cow and circulates through its bloodstream, ultimately ending up in its milk. Posi-lac (the chemical's commercial name) was approved by the Food and Drug Administration in 1993 to increase milk production despite the flooded mar-ket. The agency and Congress had been pressured by the industry to pass the hormone, although little was known about health impacts (Mills 2002). Dis-tributed first in 1994, by January 1995 Monsanto had sold 14.5 million doses (Clorfene-Casten 1996). Milk production shot up, as did the federal govern-ment's purchasing of the unconsumed, excess milk. RBGH is still being used widely used, despite experts declaring that it could be linked to cancerous growths.

Other similar debates about prevention strategies abound. Advice is often given about alcohol consumption, but, like the drunk trying to walk a straight line, science wavers in support for or against it. Evidence regarding alcohol has sometimes suggested a drink and other times claimed that it is absolutely hazardous (Smith-Warner et al. 1998). When and how many times to give birth is another question. The NCI (2003) suggests many ways in which giv-ing birth more frequently and earlier decreases risk. Yet again, this suggestion masks other factors that might be more important. Many studies that find cor-relations between giving birth and breast cancer miss a very important factor: breast-feeding.

Some research has shown that, more than giving birth, breast-feeding de-creases rates (Collaborative Group 2002; Lee et al. 2003; Heuch and Kvale 1995). The most recent studies have found that even though risk goes up the older you are when you first have a child, this risk is erased by breast-feeding (Lord et al. 2007). The most common explanation of this outcome relates to estrogen exposure in the body. Estrogen production increases breast cancer risk, but breast-feeding lowers estrogen levels. An alternative argument for why this might lower risk is that toxic chemicals that are stored in breast fat are released into milk during breast-feeding, possibly making rates go down (Patandin et al. 1999). No matter the evidence, there is still scientific dispute over the situation. The drunk continues to wobble. While these pieces of advice can be perceived as benign and important medical insight, they carry conservative and sometimes confusing overtones. For example, women have had children later generally as they have chosen to advance their educations and careers. The advice to give birth earlier suggests that they should make their careers second in importance to family.

Family history and genetics is another set of risk factors now framed as being, to some degree, within a woman's control. Women who have parents, siblings, or children with the disease; are over age sixty; or have the BRCA-1 or BRCA-2 mutation are described as "high risk" and have a set of surgical options some are beginning to take. The most radical preventive procedure is to have both breasts removed. This is a drastic measure, but to a medical community ignoring nongenetic factors, it may seem to some like the most logical option. Breast removal reduces contraction by 90 percent (Eisen and Weber 1999) and therefore seems like a reasonable option to many. However, between 20 and 70 percent of women who have the gene will never get the disease (King et al. 2003). Many prophylactic mastectomies are therefore unnecessary for the vast majority of women.

Medical advice is not benign. It has long-term, wide-ranging effects on women and their families. Urging women to follow lists of recommendations for prevention can be overwhelming and inordinate. This plethora of information makes it seem impossible to do all the right things. In addition, these trusted institutions convey breast cancer risk with false assurance. The science is controversial. Many researchers disagree that conclusions are valid.

Many scientists argue that these genetic defects are "switched" by something in the environment, like a certain type of diet or exposure to chemicals and radiation. A different set of preventive strategies would have to be employed to deal with this genetic switching. A preventive strategy taken on the basis of this knowledge would look very different than lifestyle changes. It would mandate more attention on the part of government regulators and the producers of toxins and more understanding by individual women of what could be causing breast cancer.

THE CAUSES

A victim of breast cancer loses, on average, twenty years of life (Davis 2002). She has children and, more often than not, a partner and frequently has done all the recommended things—eating fairly well, not smoking, having children before the age of thirty, and not being obese. The vast majority of the time, she does not have a family history of the disease. Even for those with one or two of these traditional risk factors, it is unlikely she will get sick. So why does breast cancer strike some women? Why are rates so high? In spite of all the research and services, there is great debate over *why* the disease is so common.

Scientists have tested many theories as to what could be causing breast cancer. There is a broad range of possibilities. Some scientists have found a promising lead that when women are exposed to too much light during the night, the circadian rhythms that regulate sleeping and waking are disrupted, leading to cancer (Sephton et al. 2000). In a recently debunked line of research, others have argued that when the surge of hormones caused by conception is prematurely ended in abortion, cellular construction is disturbed, and breast cancer risk increases (Melbye et al. 1997). Often theories that seem promising fall flat. For example, take the media frenzy over genetic mutations. The BRCA-1 and BRCA-2 mutations were linked to breast cancer in the 1990s. Immediately, newspapers, television programs, and pundits claimed that most breast cancers would soon be explained. Since then, scientists have come to realize that only a small portion is caused by family history. The promise never bore out. Like the case of genetics, some of these many theories have received more support than others. Some have been completely debunked.

One theory of causation accepted by many scientists is that the more estrogen a woman is exposed to, the higher her risk (Clark et al. 1998; Davis and Bradlow 1995). Both breast cancer research that takes biomedical approaches and that which focuses more on the environment point to the critical role of this hormone. Estrogen is actually not just one hormone but a group of them more common in women's bodies than in men's. They play a critical role in menstruation, pregnancy, and menopause. When the first two of these events take place, women are exposed to large amounts of estrogen. When a woman hits menopause, her levels decrease. There are two types of naturally occurring estrogen: the "good" and the "bad." Good estrogen is found in broccoli, other green vegetables, and soy products. Bad estrogen is that naturally coursing through the body, increasing breast cancer risk. A great deal of research has shown that bad estrogen exposure has a strong connection to the disease.

Estrogen mimics also fit into the bad category. They are a more complicated type of estrogen. Mimics are man-made chemicals whose cells take on the same shape as natural estrogen and are therefore able to make the body think it is encountering more estrogen (Sonnenschein and Soto 1998). As reflected in medical advice about breast cancer prevention, many researchers link estrogen-laden events like early menstruation, late menopause, whether you had children and when that took place, and breast-feeding with breast cancer. They even assess the usage of hormone replacement therapy. The crux of their research is that exposure to more estrogen, like that due to never giving birth or experiencing more menstrual periods, equals higher breast cancer risk.

Researchers interested in potential environmental causes study estrogens that usually exist outside the body but that get inside the body—chemicals in the environment acting as estrogens. The pivotal factor in environmental research is that chemicals that act like estrogens are just as bad as estrogen that naturally occurs in the body. Even worse, exposure to these chemicals is not circumscribed by normal life events. It can happen at any time. In fact, while naturally occurring estrogen decreases after menopause, exposure to manmade chemicals is lifelong. One such purposefully absorbed estrogen is in hormone replacement therapy, a man-made estrogen. The recent decline in breast cancer mortality has been ascribed to reduction in its use (Ravdin et al. 2007). This adds weight to the thinking that external estrogen exposure is exacerbating rates of breast cancer.

Estrogen is an important hormone in endocrine functioning. The endocrine disruptor hypothesis (EDH) is often considered the most scientifically legitimate theory that finds a link between toxic chemicals and breast cancer (Krimsky 2000). It is supported by a series of animal studies demonstrating the effect of chemicals on mammary tumor growth (Aschengrau et al. 1998). The EDH argues that the many industrial chemicals mimicking hormones from the endocrine system consequently disrupt sexual and neurological development. A growing number of researchers claim that these effects are well established and that endocrine disruptors affect breast health, which is highly subject to endocrine action. Studies show that as animals are exposed to increasing amounts of endocrine-disrupting chemicals, their development changes (Arnold et al. 1997). They may even change sex. Although this exact phenomenon is not observable in humans, cancer is.

The idea that chemicals in the environment act like human hormone changes is relatively new. Before 1992, few people suspected that chemicals in the environment might be able to enter our bodies acting as estrogen and upsetting development. Around that time, Theo Colborn, a wildlife biologist who had returned to graduate school in her sixties, began to pull different kinds of science together and saw strange overlaps in developmental defects in animals and reproductive cancers in humans. She formulated the EDH, drawing together scientists from all over the world to consider its import. Taken for its fullest ramifications, it could mean billions of dollars in lost revenues for chemical manufacturers and a complete reevaluation of today's health problems. Two of these collaborating researchers, Dr. Devra Davis and

Leon Bradlow (1995), developed and tested the idea further, then published it in *Scientific American*, where the most cutting-edge research is often first seen.

"Our proposal, based on our own research and that of others," they reported, "suggests substances we name xenoestogens (foreign estrogens) might account for some fraction of the unexplained cases" (Davis and Bradlow 1995). While estrogen is a necessary chemical in female bodies, the team argued that too much is getting into women's bloodstreams and increasing their risk. "Since World War II the amplifying varieties—found in certain pesticides, drugs, fuels and plastics—have become increasingly prevalent in modern societies," they explained. The short and concise article emerged in 1995 to a mixed reception of scientific incredulity and celebration. Since then, endocrine-disrupting chemicals have still been brought to market.

Such chemicals permeate the planet, but exposures can also be location based. Breast cancer rates are not consistent across the United States or around the world. Geography shapes incidence, like power shapes prevention and race determines outcomes. There are pockets of the United States where breast cancer cases have risen six times faster than other areas (Clarke et al. 2002). The worst areas are the industrialized regions where power plants, refineries, and manufacturing facilities pump toxic particles into the air and wastewater into local streams (Kulldorff et al. 1997). The pesticide load of modern agriculture may also contribute to rising breast cancer rates since many of the chemicals routinely sprayed on fruits and vegetables are linked to cancer (Davis et al. 1993). Places where these exposures aggregate often bear witness to some of the highest rates of the illness.

There are hot spots around the country that reflect these patterns of chemicals. Marin County, California, has the highest breast cancer rates in the world (Northern California Cancer Center 1994). Long Island, New York, has rates ranging up to 200 percent over the national average (New York State Department of Public Health 1999). The rates at Cape Cod, Massachusetts, are at least 20 percent higher than the national average (Silent Spring Institute 1998). All these places were the site of long-term agriculture and industry, now reclaimed for the rich.

Cape Cod was long the site of potato farming for Portuguese immigrants. It later became home to endless red seas of cranberry bogs. Those crops require pesticide spraying that, after passing over burgeoning young plants, leaches into the groundwater, then returns to homes in wells and city water. Extensive studies are now being done on the cape, and researchers have found that women are exposed to a long list of chemicals, many of which were used long ago but remain in their carpets, dust, and yards. Could it be that the pesticides applied over the years on Cape Cod, in addition to cleaning products meant to control the sea mold, have driven breast cancer rates up to what they are today?

⌒∕⌒

West Islip, Long Island, is now a commuter community for New York City, but not so long ago it was an agricultural and fishing town. Set on the Long Island Sound, oyster boats once clogged its marinas, culling an abundant ocean harvest most days of the season. When the Dutch arrived hundreds of years ago, they turned Long Island into a farming haven for lettuce, tomatoes, beets, parsley, corn, herbs, and especially potatoes. Those days are long past. Today, the oyster boats are gone, and farmers have vanished. Women with breast cancer remain. Their bodies are the fleshy witnesses of industry once here, now erased except in its fallout.

Robin moved into her house on Secataug Lane with her husband, Eddy, thirteen years ago. Prior to that, she lived in another town on the south shore of Long Island, a little closer to New York City. Both areas have high rates of breast cancer.

"He feels guilty for living here," Robin explains about Eddy, who grew up in their boxlike four-bedroom cottage in West Islip. The couple moved in when they first got married and before Robin gave birth to her first child at the age of thirty-two. In response to her comment, Eddy stares into the distance, a hedge next to the inlet where several of his boats are for sale. His business—and the ease of moving back home—has pulled them to this area. Sitting on the back porch in the late afternoon, this place seems idyllic, far from home to tragedy.

"We are going to make it through this. Everything is going to be fine," is his slower-than-normal response. They sit talking about what is going to happen the following morning. They will go to the hospital, where she will have a bilateral mastectomy. Cancerous growth was found only in Robin's left breast, but it was the kind of cancer that often moves to the other. And so she decided to have them both removed and replaced by new implants.

"The idea would have been disgusting to me, if it weren't my wife," said Eddy. "Neither me nor Robin knows how we're gonna feel when the surgery is done."

"But there is no other way to go. I want them off," Robin pushed in response. She looked at me, then away. Neither of them spoke. The whispering breeze swept past the pool and out onto the canal it overlooked. Silence was marked by the lack of children's voices, the lack of Robin's chatter, and the emptiness of Robin's and Eddy's fear.

Robin is one of thousands of women who will have the same experience this year—no family history, no reason to worry, and complete surprise when the lump is biopsied and the cancer is diagnosed.

CHANGING THE DEBATE

The initial approach to breast cancer was finding it and treating it. This subsumes a huge amount of resources and is still vastly important. But the need for prevention has been obscured by more than narrow-mindedness. It is also about purposeful ignorance. Vested interests like large chemical manufacturers and governmental regulators, congressmen, and presidents they back are hard pressed to look squarely at how their actions could be causing the disease. There is much to lose. Breast cancer is not a conspiracy; it is hypocrisy. Changing the debate depends on corporate transparency, government accountability, and public transformation.

Chemicals in daily products, chlorinated drinking water, hormones in food, pesticides, and a vast array of other toxic exposures are factors largely ignored by the largest funders of research like the National Institute of Health, the National Cancer Society, and pharmaceutical companies. However, these factors may promise to reveal answers about the illness. Millions of new research dollars, a sprinkling of advocacy groups, and several attentive politicians are making a growing case that such environmental factors are important. They claim that the popular representation of breast cancer prevention is based only on one body of scientific evidence, the majority of which is funded by vested interests like the pharmaceutical industry. Some scientists and advocates also point out that research is far from objective and that what gets publicized often leaves out a great deal of important evidence.

"There is a huge imbalance in resources between corporate science and public interest science," argues Dr. Julia Brody, director of the Silent Spring Institute, the only research group devoted solely to studying potential environmental causes of breast cancer. "It just hadn't crossed my mind that breast cancer research was being driven by patents. Patents for genetic tests, for pharmaceuticals, for new mammography machines."

This drive for profit rather than prevention has led to a predominant disregard for environmental toxins. This is one of the blatant shortcomings of the "war on cancer." Carcinogenic industrial chemicals came into major production after World War II as the economic boom fueled the production of chemicals and synthetics that had proved critical in battle. Dr. Ana Soto from Tufts University points out that "the increasing risk of breast cancer and other cancers has paralleled the proliferation of synthetic chemicals since World War

II." The ineffective testing of these chemicals before public consumption has resulted in their possessing some level of carcinogenicity (Colborn et al. 1993). On average, Americans have more than fifty chemicals linked to illness coursing through their blood, being stored in fat cells and visitors in tissue (Centers for Disease Control and Prevention 2003). We consume food that has been sprayed with them, use beauty products that contain them, and clean our houses with products replete with these chemicals. Science has shown these products to cause cancer, and our exposure to them increases as we fill our gas tanks with them, spray them onto our lawns, and brush them onto our eyelids and nails.

Like breast cancer itself, exposure to chemicals and the possible ramifications thereof seem unthreatening—distant and safe. Unlike my own experience where I can remember one toxic chemical that I was exposed to as a child, many of us have little awareness of what we have absorbed or inhaled. We can probably recall diving into the cool blue water of the neighborhood pool as a child and the pungent chlorine odor that accompanied us home. Few of us knew that, like a long list of chemicals in products we use on a daily basis, chlorine is carcinogenic and that our cumulative exposure to it in drinking water and food and during summer afternoons could be make us sick, not just cool (Bernard et al. 2006).

In addition to our own ignorance of possibly harmful exposures, there are economic reasons for ignoring environmental causes of breast cancer. Large corporations with major financial stakes in treatment regimens and detection devices are loathe to put any attention toward prevention, and, even more, many industries that are the source of toxic exposures actively lobby and campaign against better regulations (Stauber and Rampton 1995). In the case of breast cancer, many activists have been unwittingly brought into campaigns leading down the road away from a cause and instead into more and more breast cancer.

Chapter Two

How We Got Here

Man can hardly even recognize the evils of his own creation.

—Albert Schweitzer

The afternoon was winding down, and Robin and Eddy needed to get things ready before she would go to the hospital the next morning. Eddy was worried about Robin and about the cost. But he wouldn't let Robin or the kids see that if he could help it. It was the middle of his biggest season, and he could not tell how it would shake out in terms of how many boats he could sell. Sales were hard to make. If he was going to send the kids to summer camp and keep on schedule with renovating the house, he was going to have to hold it together.

Little Eddy was the youngest and so understood the least. He was six. Even at that age, he was the spitting image of his father: round brown eyes and olive skin, a straight nose, and high cheekbones. His personality was just a generation behind his father's. Big Eddy is energetic, always walking briskly, often ahead of the kids. His speech matches his body, an undulating tone highlighting his otherwise gentle Long Island accent. Little Eddy is years away from the little calm his father had earned with time, his energy nervous and unrelenting. His mouth could barely keep up with his thoughts as he tripped over words and pushed through sentences he was almost too impatient to finish. He was not yet ready to understand what was happening to his mother. Robin said she had a stomachache. But he knew something was wrong, even though he did not have the words to express it.

The two girls were boundlessly curious and talkative like Little Eddy but more mature. Tori was ten, and Brittany, who was Robin's younger twin, was twelve. Both were old enough to be uncomfortable about discussing breasts but young enough to be incapable of grasping the idea of breasts being re-moved. I asked them how they felt about their mom's operation. They both giggled quietly and turned away, not answering clearly. Later, they might try to understand, but now it seemed that fear was masked by a hidden and in-tense need for Mom to be okay.

FOUR WAVES OF ACTIVISM: MAKING AND BREAKING THE POLITICAL ECONOMY

Activism has put breast cancer into the public's eye, at the same time associ-ating the disease with cure and treatment, mammography, and hope. This public portrayal relates directly to the movement's relationship with large corporations producing treatments and detection devices. This political econ-omy of activism has guided advocacy educational events in a way that devel-ops more attention for pharmaceutical products and for detection. While breast cancer activism has driven more research and awareness, it is impor-tant to ask, What has driven the movement?

The first wave of breast cancer activism began with Rose Kushner, Bab-bette Rosomond, and the few women who took the risk to tell their story to the public (Batt 1995; Rosenbaum and Roos 2000). These women opened a new door for awareness, support, and the subsequent legacy of courageous activists. The second wave arose as support groups and the first breast cancer organizations formed, drawing attention to the massive number of cases, the need for better treatment, and the necessity of assistance from families and friends (Altman 1996). This wave established the public perception of breast cancer that continues today—a message of awareness, need for progress, and hope for women with breast cancer. Then and now, progress was centered around detection, treatment, and cure, an essential purpose for women who, at that time, needed many challenges in these areas. This message seems sim-ple, straightforward, and unquestionable. But there are many other ways that breast cancer can be presented, and there are reasons why it has maintained this image even when there is plenty of awareness, many needs are being met, and hope is not the only feeling that surrounds these efforts.

There is an explanation why breast cancer public education has not changed much from its founding days. Money may be the most important. At the same time these organizations were founded, large corporations devel-oped simultaneous or even overlapping education campaigns. Although cor-porate support of nonprofits is typical (Shamir 2004) and sometimes even necessary, an ethical dilemma plagues this case. The most involved corpora-tions profit from increased demand for detection devices and treatment regimens. Others accrue massive profits from pinning a gendered, philanthropic cause to their name while actually contributing to toxic exposures linked with breast cancer risk. These large businesses fund activism, education campaigns, and the largest proportion of breast cancer research. As a result, they have shaped how the public understands the disease and the topics of much research. In this way, the political economy of breast cancer is also a political economy of social movements, of activism, and of social change.

The first campaigns by these corporations with vested interests led to other corporations joining what had become the many groups involved in the second wave of breast cancer activism. Each new corporation and group built on the last, generally with only slight variation. The trajectory of these efforts had an inertia that was difficult to interrupt. Sociologists have given this a somewhat convoluted name—institutional isomorphism. They argue that organizations tend to become more and more like one another rather than diversify (DiMaggio and Powell 1983). In part, this is due to the uncertainty of breaking out of current patterns. It is much easier for managers and directors to follow the tried-and-true path than to generate new ones. And it is safer too.

Training of professionals plays a part in this process. For example, as scientists go through similar classes and work on related research projects, they end up repeating the same methods and pursuing similar questions. Even in companies where presidents attempt to restructure in order to be more competitive, the constraints of expectations, values, and "normal" methods hinder this process. In practice, for breast cancer, this means that profits from breast cancer drugs and detection devices, pink products to support research or a sick friend, and research funding from corporations all lead back to the same focus—treatment, detection, and cure.

The establishment of detection, treatment, and cure as the predominant approach makes investigating causes a risk for scientists. Their methods and tools are less well-established, and there are far fewer funds available to support their work (Brown et al. 2006). Their results can also pose serious challenges to very powerful corporations whose public relations experts and scientific advisory boards can spend endless dollars discrediting science they do not like. Few scientists are willing to build a career around such a dicey field.

These first two waves of breast cancer activism were followed by two more that have reshaped the political economy of breast cancer yet again. The third wave pushed through funding for new research and governmental support, making breast cancer more political yet noncontroversial. The fourth wave, focused on causation, has stripped away this face of breast cancer to reveal corporate malfeasance, denial, suffering, and a new paradigm of illness. Following the trajectories of these waves of activism tells the story of breast cancer's changing political and scientific economy.

THE FIRST VOICES

While institutions and professions now structure the individual experiences of millions of women, the story of how we arrived here begins instead with a few brave women who shared their experiences with the public. I began encountering their voices under dim lights in the hushed, marble Boston Public Library. One of the earliest projects I worked on when I started graduate school was a paper about how the media portrayed breast cancer. I was looking as far back as the 1960s when the cover of the *Ladies Home Journal* featured meatloaf and Jackie O. I pulled magazines from deep in the library archives up until the present day, where articles had already been archived online. Initially I could not believe I had gone to graduate school to do this grunt work, weeks of photocopying and stapling. I flipped through old but crisp copies of *Good Housekeeping*, *Ladies Home Journal*, *Glamour*, *Vogue*, and every other women's and newsmagazine possible. While standing over the flashing lights of the copy machine, I became fascinated by the magazines as both a time machine back to another decade and a reflection of how little we have changed apart from hemlines and hat styles.

The women writers whose work filled the pages told the story of how breast cancer began to enter the public consciousness. One of the crucial events, appropriately covered by most publications, was reported when Happy Rockefeller came out of the closet about her experience with the disease. Even in the 1970s, cancer was a silent killer. It was hidden behind hospital doors, unknown to children, only whispered among friends. Happy was the first public figure to put her face on the pages of magazines. A few images portrayed her lying in a bed of white sheets, smiling and energetic. Under the covers, her breasts seemed to be intact. Most of the photographs did not go behind the scenes but showed her with her husband, Senator Nelson Rockefeller, waving at crowds, triumphant over cancer. Similar to her story was First Lady Betty Ford, who was next to publicize the radical surgery she underwent in 1974 and emerged seemingly cured.

Happy and Betty started a trend. Books about the breast cancer experience began to fill bookstore shelves, and women started to use these monographs to understand what they could expect and how they could deal with the disease (Batt 1995). In the 1980s, support groups began to form. That was the first time cancer's shame was removed and the problems it caused with sex, family, and money were openly discussed. These circles contained secrets and deep friendships. This camaraderie blossomed into breast cancer organizations determined to get better treatment options for women and to generate more awareness about the disease to increase chances of survival. Throughout the 1980s, the first stage of breast cancer activism was forming

(Casamayou 2001). Groups that supplied information and assistance to women blossomed and support groups became common (Gardner 2006). Women began to see themselves as part of a community.

For the first time in American history, these women attacked the sexism of the health research system in the United States. They pushed forward the need to address women's health issues, facing the shroud of secrecy around women's stigmatized vaginas and breasts, and changing the "otherness" of women's health into a mainstream, marketable area of research. These groups became political. They helped instigate new policies, including the succession of bills passed in the early 1990s under President Clinton.

The Mammography Quality Standards Act of 1992 mandated that mammography facilities follow strict regulations about the quality of their services (Weisman 2000; Zones 2000). This was followed by the first major breast cancer–specific policy called the President's Plan on Breast Cancer in 1993 (Steingraber 2000). It laid out an agenda for research, public education, access, and health care regulation. The 1997 Stamp Out Breast Cancer Act was the first disease-specific stamp (King 2006). By 2005, it generated more than $40 million. Proceeds go to the National Institutes of Health and the Department of Defense.

State policies grew up with federal support. The first major policy to offer government funding to cover mammography or breast cancer screening was the 1988 Medicare Catastrophic Coverage Act, which was a direct result of letter writing and organizing put together by Rose Kushner (Casamayou 2001). Two years later, the federal Breast and Cervical Cancer Prevention Act was passed to help low-income and uninsured women get access to screening (Brenner 2000). Many states have chosen to augment the Medicaid funding that the federal government offered by passing breast and cervical health programs or acts. Most of these policies focused on access to mammography and basic biological research.

I learned about more and more organizations that popped up. They raised vast sums of money for support services and began getting research into treatment and cure. At that time, the government had done little.

One of the first and most powerful was the Susan G. Komen Foundation. Wealthy and polished Nancy Brinker founded it in 1981 when her sister died of the disease. As Brinker relates the story, her sister Suzy was diagnosed at age thirty-two. In recovery, she said from her hospital bed, "Nan, if Mrs. Ford can admit she has breast cancer and tell the whole world she intends to fight it, well then so can I" (Komen 2007a). She was waiting for her first chemotherapy treatment despite the doctors declaring her cured five months prior. New examinations had shown that the cancer had spread under her arm and in her lungs. But it was 1978 in Peoria, Illinois. Treatment was poor. Nine operations, three courses of chemotherapy and radiation, and three years later, Suzy died.

Doctors found lumps in Nan's breasts, but they were benign. Nan lived on. Inspired by her sister, she created one of the largest breast cancer foundations in the world. It provides services to women with breast cancer far beyond decorating the walls of their hospital rooms. Being the head of such an organization led Nan into an elite social world to become the ambassador to Hungary and a close friend of high-profile fashion designers, chief executive officers of makeup companies, and pharmaceutical giants. In the mid-1990s, Komen garnered a little under $50 million annually, and by the early twenty-first century, the foundation was raising slightly less than $140 million every year (Komen for the Cure 2007b).

Few other breast cancer organizations had formed in the early 1980s. The disease was under wraps. The American Cancer Society (ACS) helped keep its effects undercover by sponsoring programs such as Reach for Recovery and Look Good, Feel Good. While they provided limited, one-on-one support from women who previously had breast cancer (Love and Lindsey 1997), they were focused primarily on returning women to a feminine beauty standard by encouraging them to wear temporary breast prostheses and put on makeup every day. This disguising of breast cancer was partially in response to the social stigmatization of the disease. Strong cultural perceptions of the breast as related to vitality, sexuality, and motherhood kept people quiet. It was not just a threat to one's health but also to one's femininity.

Slowly, over that decade, other organizations of all sizes arose—small local groups provided services, and large groups, like the National Association of Breast Cancer Organizations, provided information. Some spoke out publicly about breast cancer to denounce the shame surrounding the disease (Anglin 1997; Casamayou 2001). This was the second wave of activism. It was courageous and groundbreaking. But early on, these organizations had to raise money. That need would change the face of breast cancer for good.

CORPORATIZING ACTIVISM

In 1984, the executive directors of Imperial Chemical Incorporated (ICI), Cancer Care Inc., and the American Association of Cancer Care Physicians met to discuss the growing breast cancer crisis and how to educate Americans about detection and treatment. More and more women seemed to be succumbing to the disease, but few were using mammography, the only medical test for detection. In addition, the company had taken a turn for the worse in the late 1970s thanks to overinvestment in petrochemicals, plastics, and agricultural goods. It reported that even after reorganizing and streamlining, it had to "make greater levels of profitability and market penetration, and change its product profile" (Pettigrew 1985). Pharmaceuticals were the next venture, and it would need a consumer base. The tripartite combined tremendous resources. Cancer Care Inc. provided services: hotlines, information about how to tell kids the news, support groups, and educational programs. The Association of Cancer Care Physicians represented a quickly expanding group of professionals, and ICI provided financial support for the project.

In 1998, ICI gave birth to AstraZeneca, a company that would have long-term effects on breast cancer. The crew team rowing serenely and forcefully across a seamless artificial blue sea on the front of the company's annual report is reminiscent of inspirational posters that propose, "There is no I in TEAM." The company's $18.8 billion sales figure is as unbelievable as the azure deep across which the AstraZeneca team glides. It employs 2,000 people conducting research and development at eleven different centers, including the director of the board, David Brennan, who grossed $4,865,000 in 2006 and chief financial officer Jonathan Symons, who made the second most at $2,149,000 that same year (AstraZeneca 2006). Seven countries host facilities: Sweden, the United Kingdom, the United States, Canada, France, India, and Japan. Manufacturing is even larger. Fourteen thousand workers support twenty-seven manufacturing sites in nineteen countries. Sales for AstraZeneca in 2004 totaled $21.4 billion. Forty-five percent of that was in the United States, 36 percent in Europe, 6 percent in Japan, and 13 percent in the rest of the world. Around the globe, there were a total of 60,000 employees (AstraZeneca 2004).

The seeming stability and profit of such a large venture is entirely dependent on a gamble—what will be consumed at the greatest rate? This question is in turn dependent on two others—what drug will work the best, and what kind of marketing can be used to encourage consumers to buy it? In other words, the company must be closely attuned to patterns of consumption and to innovation in marketing. Being attentive to these trends is the only way to manage the high stakes of breast cancer drug development and promotion.

Millions of dollars are invested in research and development of new drugs and even more for marketing before any proceeds are returned to the company (Angell 2004). New products present tremendous risk. The company acknowledges, "Patients respond differently to different therapies," so there is open competition for the consumption of these drugs. Like any private enterprise, patenting is important. But as the AstraZeneca website claims, "Patents do not create a monopoly for treating a disease—other manufacturers are able to develop a different medicine to treat the same condition. Also, patents are limited in time and after their expiration, competitors (both innovative and generic) can legitimately market the same product" (http://www.astrazeneca.com). This marketing is critical. Bringing the consumer to the product leads to financial returns on the millions spent on research and development. AstraZeneca is like most other pharmaceutical companies in its major investment in marketing. In 2004, the company spent $7.84 billion in that department, about twice as much as it spent on research and development (Ismail 2006).

Since many of AstraZeneca's breast cancer drugs depend on spotting the disease early enough so that a woman can use it for a lengthy period after diagnosis, catching it early is important. Mammography has been the key to early diagnosis since the 1960s. The high-level financial risks taken on drug development and the growing potential for using mammography as a main screening tool is enough motivation for AstraZeneca to promote treatment and detection. The company, with its two team members, created National Breast Cancer Awareness Month (NBCAM) as an event to educate women about these options and increase awareness. In this case, greater awareness means a bigger market.

These collaborators represented cutting-edge activism. Their event was one of the first on a national level to create breast cancer awareness. The innovation, novelty, and groundbreaking work of founding such an event meant that the team could shape the public image of what to do about the disease. They could tell people how to regain a sense of control and how to make the disease go away. The three-part team designed the event, and AstraZeneca copyrighted it. The company offers downloads on its website so that any other organization can use its symbols and graphics. At the same time, however, owning the copyright means that if someone uses the trademark in a way the company deems inappropriate, then it can be stopped or even sued (Graphic Artist's Guild 2006). The company actually holds approval privileges over the usage of the trademark (Paulsen 1993), meaning that AstraZeneca controls the image, messages, and outcomes of NBCAM.

The debate about corporate funding has raged among breast cancer organizations. It is far from clear what is ethical and what is not. While some advocates justify the involvement of corporations by explaining that they have no other source of funding or that their activities are not influenced by the funder, others claim that these arguments are far from sound. Barron Lerner, professor of medicine at Columbia University, argues that such organizations are reminiscent of doctors who are wined and dined, educated, and paid by drug companies, but who still argue that their opinion is professionally independent. Columbia, like many other medical schools, is debating how to get rid of corporate influence over research. Controversy has raged over whether experts can maintain independence when, for example, they are invited to musicals and supplied plane tickets and hotels to attend conferences on the splendid French Riviera, as AstraZeneca recently did (Boseley 2006).

While a corporation's motives are questioned for doing something like this, they are simultaneously congratulated for giving similar resources to breast cancer groups. What is missed in this equation is that consumers and patients get as much information from nonprofit educational programs as they do from doctors. In fact, many individuals already know what drug they want before they see their doctor (Brodie 2001). About 50 percent of the time when a patient requests a particular drug, she gets it (Mintzes et al. 2002). Breast cancer organizations that piggyback on corporate funding or corporate events may be convinced to buy into an agenda that they themselves did not create and that may not be in their best interests. It sounds innocent enough that pharmaceutical companies want to help find a "cure." We forget or overlook that it is to their financial benefit. In the meantime, other, possibly more productive research topics could be pursued that might improve quality of life.

Since its inception, NBCAM has grown to be the most widely known breast cancer event in America. Major government agencies, foundations, professional medical organizations, and nonprofits take part in publicizing it, including the National Cancer Institute, the ACS, the American College of Radiology, and CancerCare, among others (NBCAM 2007). Organizers make their agenda clear. The informational brochure says, "In an effort to encourage women to have an annual mammography screening, National Breast Cancer Awareness Month (NBCAM) sponsors recommend making every day National Mammography Day." Event sponsors do not pretend to promote any other tool.

Pressure to get mammograms has grown with the national expansion of the event. Even the former president of the United States is a supporter. In 2003, President Bush made a commitment: "I . . . do hereby proclaim the month of October 2003 as National Breast Cancer Awareness Month. I call upon Government officials, businesses, communities, healthcare professionals, educators, volunteers, and all the people of the United States to continue our Nation's strong commitment to controlling and curing breast cancer."

Barbara Brenner, director of the group Breast Cancer Action, claimed that because of AstraZeneca's dependency on treatment profits, "you will just not see any information about prevention" at an NBCAM event sponsored by the company. "It just won't happen." Brenner argues that there is too much at stake in potential profits for the company to direct any support toward causes. Additionally, AstraZeneca, like most large manufacturing facilities, has good reason to draw attention away from environmental causes in particular. AstraZeneca has a history of dumping toxic chemicals linked to cancer and not cleaning up (Batt and Gross 1999; Dow Jones Business Wire 2000). Zeneca, one of the two companies that joined to form AstraZeneca, is the third-largest polluter in Britain, dumping the same toxics into the environment that remain in women's breasts (Arlidge 1999).

Similar problems have occurred in the United States. The federal government and the state of California have sued AstraZeneca for toxic dumping. GB Biosciences, a subsidiary of AstraZeneca that produces pesticides, was sued by the city of Houston in 2002 for $6.1 million after it allowed chemicals to flow into the soil, groundwater, and a local bayou. The plant operating adjacent to a functioning port had been manufacturing chemicals there for fifty years, slowly allowing contaminants to leach into the ground (Hensel 2002). AstraZeneca and ICI have a financial interest in diverting political attention away from the importance of better regulating polluting chemicals that their facilities emit. They have an additional interest in keeping the movement focused on treatment since this focus means that there will be a market for their products.

Brenner is perhaps one of the first to name the process through which companies simultaneously produce carcinogenic chemicals and curative pharmaceuticals. She calls it the "the cancer industry" (personal communication, 2006). She uses that term to describe AstraZeneca, Avon, Estée Lauder, Ford Motors, and many other companies whose products are toxic but whose philanthropic goals include eradicating the disease. With focus directed to detection and cure, there is no conflict of interest for these companies. They can pollute and put money into curative pharmaceuticals. Placing the emphasis on prevention would radically change this situation. Companies would have to use nontoxic chemicals in production. Drugs would be truly preventive, working toward decreasing rates of breast cancer, not just decreasing death rates. But as Devra Davis, who coined the term "xenoestrogens" and whose center at Carnegie Mellon University researches causes of cancer, says, "The economic incentives for preventing breast cancer are not there. There is a lot more to be made from treating breast cancer than preventing it right now (Davis, personal communication, 2007).

THE GOVERNMENT ON DRUGS?

Not only have AstraZeneca and other corporations bought the public perception of breast cancer, but they also work hand in hand with the government. This process can involve the most straightforward form—lobbying—or, less obviously, state agencies using tax dollars to benefit large pharmaceutical companies. A recent document from the Center for Public Integrity in Washington, D.C., reports that in the past seven years the pharmaceutical industry has spent more than $800 million on federal and state lobbying campaigns (Ismail 2006). These companies target a multitude of government agencies, including Congress, the Department of Health and Human Services, the Food and Drug Administration, and the State Department. About $133 million takes the form of campaign contributions, while other amounts go to supporting staffers working for congressmen or donations.

This type of government influence is well known. Less obvious is the way that government programs and tax dollars result in major gains for pharmaceutical interests. Take the National Institutes of Health (NIH). It dedicates a huge amount of money to cancer research, most of which is used for the very basics of research, like the cellular functioning of the disease. Since finding a cure or treatment depends first on understanding this biological function, large pharmaceutical companies depend on it. As Dr. Marcia Angell, former editor of the *New England Journal of Medicine*, describes, the federal government frequently develops a way to treat a disease, but since it is a nonprofit institution, it cannot sell it. Therefore, the government sells the patent to a company that will market and distribute a drug. In the process, the company makes a huge profit. An example of this is Taxol, a drug manufactured by Bristol-Myers Squibb but researched and developed by researchers at the NIH. The company paid the NIH $35 million for the patent, then proceeded to make $9 billion in sales (Angell 2004)—certainly a hefty return on investment.

The professional practices and training of researchers also facilitate support for large pharmaceutical companies. While medical schools depend on pharmaceutical funding to conduct research, such support also influences the kind of work they do and the type of training they provide. All this adds up to the fact that academic researchers, government workers, or individuals who slide back and forth between these different worlds do much of the research that pharmaceutical corporations use for their products (Krimsky 2003). This facile process means that the types of research done will be similar across sectors. As a result, money continues to be invested in profitable research trajectories rather than topics that might actually challenge industries.

CAUSE MARKETING

While many companies may come to mind when you think about breast cancer—Yoplait, Kellogg's, or even the U.S. Postal Service—AstraZeneca would not be one of them. While AstraZeneca was possibly the first corporation to sponsor breast cancer philanthropy, a range of corporations that previously had nothing to do with breast cancer followed. They recognized a growing market niche: women who had breast cancer along with their very concerned friends or family members. Corporations profit from these groups through new products—teddy bears, bracelets, T-shirts, pillows, purses, and a vast array of items—or through increasing sales for a label that looks philanthropic. Some of these products have something to do with the illness, and others can just be given as gifts. It seems an odd idea at best to give someone who has undergone a mastectomy or months of chemotherapy a pink purse that reminds her of the ordeal every time she picks it up and goes to work. Somehow, though, these products have become popularized.

Many of these items are used for "cause marketing." Companies joined the breast cancer fight with cause marketing in the early 1990s. Through it, nonprofit organizations can partner with a corporation to raise money. The corporation funds the advertising for a certain organization or event, and in turn for its help, an organization receives a portion of proceeds. By 2004, consumer spending on cause marketing in the United States was estimated to be around $988 million (Cause Marketing Forum 2003). The advantage is that these funds are often more than the organization could raise on its own. The disadvantage is that consumers fill the gap left by decreases in governmental social welfare policies. They are now the key to supporting the downtrodden or needy through spending.

Breast cancer groups have become experts at cause marketing. Possibly the most practiced breast cancer organization is the Komen Foundation. Nancy Brinker, who heads the foundation, began cause marketing in the early 1990s when most disease-based groups had not even thought of it. One of their early campaigns was with Ford Motors. At first, the slogan was "Committed to the Cause," then "Tied to the Cause," with sales of a scarf that women tied around their necks in advertisements in major women's magazines. During this campaign, Ford, the Komen Foundation, and various retail outlets sold a breast cancer scarf, and the profit from the sales went to the Komen Foundation. By 2005, scarf sales totaled $1,645,490, with 85 percent going to Komen (Komen 2007c). Sheryl Crow, Susan Sarandon, Cuba Gooding Jr., Kirsten Dunst, Katie Holmes, Pete Sampras, Sarah Michelle Gellar, Helen Hunt, Serena Williams, Courtney Cox, David Arquette, Vanessa Williams, and Renée Zellweger have helped promote Ford's Tied to the Cause campaign. These actors, singer/songwriters, and athletes have posed in high-profile print ads wearing the Ford scarf. Ford also encourages its employees to participate in Race for the Cure events across the country. As of 2006, the company has dedicated more than $87 million to the foundation in donations and in-kind gifts (http://www.ford.com).

Komen has also had many other cause-marketing sponsors: Yoplait, whose Save Lids to Save Lives campaign makes around $1.2 million a year, and Deluxe Company's Checks for the Cure, which raised $530,000 in 2000. According to an interview between a Komen Foundation representative and Cindy Schneible from Cause Marketing Forum (Schneible 2003),

> Komen partners with companies whose commitment to the breast cancer cause is significant and clearly disclosed to consumers. [In 2002] we had approximately 60 partners. Some of the largest are Lee Jeans, for Lee National Denim Day; Yoplait which runs the Save Lids to Save Lives program and is the national presenting sponsor of the Komen Race for the Cure Series; BMW North America for the Ultimate Drive promotion; and the Women's International Bowling Congress which runs the Bowl for a Cure programs.

Komen is not the only group that has built an excellent cause marketing campaign. The Breast Cancer Research Foundation has partnered with Target to create a pink bull's-eye. The company even set up a temporary store in Times Square to sell breast cancer products. In that case, all proceeds from the products went directly to the foundation. Other campaigns include several financial companies, like American Express's Charge for the Cure, where American Express gives a much smaller amount, 1 percent of a purchase, to research; Charles Schwab's Commission for the Cure; and Kinetics Asset Management Medical Fund's Invest for the Cure. A range of other stores also promote causes, like Hallmark's Cards for the Cure, Goldsmith Seeds's Plant for the Cure, and Lee Jeans National Denim Day "Wear Denim for the Cure." Lee Jeans has raised $44 million for Komen (Komen 2007b) (see table 2.1).

Cause marketing appears to be a win–win situation. The public sees the corporation as a worthwhile investment: a philanthropist. Sales go up. The collaborating organization makes some money too. But critics of cause marketing argue that the for-profit organization involved has more to gain than the nonprofit. Frequently, only a small portion of the money used to purchase a particular product goes to the cause that it publicizes. This is true of many of Komen's campaigns. Around 10 percent of their Cook for the Cure products goes to the foundation, while the rest goes to the manufacturer.

Other corporate partners have a conflict of interest with funding breast cancer research in particular. For example, Ford Motors has a vested interest in profits from car sales. However, research has found that chemicals in car exhaust are linked with increased breast cancer risk (Gammon et al. 2002a). Therefore, partnering with Ford could lead activism away from preventing the illness. Ford Division has acted as the national series sponsor of the Susan G. Komen Foundation Race for the Cure for the past twelve years. Similarly,

Table 2.1. Sampling of Product Campaigns for Susan G. Komen Foundation

Product/Campaign	Amt Per Purchase	Total $ Raised	Total to Komen	Years
Cook for the cure	*	$4 million	*	2001–2006
Mixer	$319.99	$50	*	
Mixer cover	$29.99	$2.99	*	
Toaster	$69.99	$7.00	*	
Silicone heart-shaped cookware	$15.99	$1.59	*	
Glass pitcher	$129.99	$10	*	
Polycarbonate pitcher	$129.99	$10	*	
Coffee mill	$129.99	$10	*	
Teapot	$9.99	$5	*	
Peeler	$10.99	$1.09	*	
Ice cream scoop	$14.99	$1.49	*	
Spatula	$14.99	$1.49	*	
Whisk	$14.99	$1.49	*	
Satoku knife	$14.99	$1.49	*	
Measuring cups & Spoons	$9.99	$.99	*	
Can Opener	$19.99	$1.99	*	
Scissors	$19.99	$1.99	*	
Santoku knife	$24.99	42.49	*	
Food processor	$249.99	$25.00	*	
Hand mixer	$79.99	$7.00	*	
Kitchen hand towel	$19.95	$5.00	*	
4-piece kitchen towel set	$39.99	$5.00	*	
Tomboy Tools– Hammer out Breast Cancer	$14.95	$6.00	Guaranteed 100,000	2006–2007
Oreck- Clean for the Cure Vacuum Cleaner	$549.00	$50	Guaranteed 250,000	2006–2007
US Bowling Congress –Roll Breast Cancer into the Gutter		1 cent/pin at specific events	$4 million	2001–2006
American Airlines		*	5.7 million	1992–2006
BMW–The Ultimate Drive		$1 per mile	9 million	1997–2006

Product/Campaign	Amt Per Purchase	Total $ Raised	Total to Komen	Years
The Carslile Collection	*	Each $125 donation gets a scarf	1 million	1998–2006
Ford Division–Race for the Cure Sponsor	*	*	*	1994–2006
Ford Division Warriors for the Cure	40–80% of apparel proceeds	*	3.5 million	2002–2006
Hallmark Gold Crown Stores	9.95 Olivia Newton John CD & ornament	$2	Guaranteed 100,000	2006
Kellogg Company– Help Unlock the Cure	*	$5 for 2 cereal box UPC symbols	*	2001–2006
Lean Cuisine–Do Something Good for the Cure	*	10 cents per dinner	1 million	2001–2006
The Val Skinner Foundation–LGPA LIFE Event	*		1.5 million	2000–2006
M&Ms	*	35 or 50 cents per package	Guaranteed 250,000	2006
Mowhawk Industries Decorate for the Cure	*	10 cents per yard	1.3 million	2001–2006

Note: The information in this table was drawn from http://cms.komen.org/komen/Partners/CorporatePartners/index.htm.
* Information unavailable.

Komen has received in-kind donations from companies with which it might have a conflict of interest, like Occidental Chemical Corporation, which supplies its office space and is also a member of its Million Dollar Council (Cause Marketing Forum 2003).

Possibly the most important critique of cause marketing is the most difficult to substantiate. When the public is trained to buy for a cure or spend money to support women with breast cancer, they come to believe that have participated in improving the situation and the lives of women. This monetary participation replaces a more meaningful engagement with the issue by learning about it and making a commitment to changing it. Buying is a quick fix, immediate gratification, and consumerism at its best. But it does little to prevent the epidemic.

Criticisms of cause marketing have arisen from many groups. The point is not to stop fund-raising for cancer. The point is to change the way it works. Consumers can learn to be more careful about where their dollars go. With this, the marketer of the cause brings in funds because it is really doing something people care about, not simply because it has tied the corporate name to breast cancer. On the other hand, the recipients of cause-marketing dollars can take the initiative to invest the money diversely—possibly into prevention as well as treatment and cure.

When I arrived at Robin's house early the next morning, a new car was in the driveway. She was borrowing her mother's car for a few weeks, a silver Mercedes coupe—just big enough for the kids but not frumpy. It fit her. I pulled past the driveway and noticed a bright flash of color as I passed and parked my car on the street. Walking to the house, I realized that a pink ribbon had been pasted onto the back of the car. It seemed trivial, but its significance struck me. She was no longer a sympathizer. She was one of tens of thousands of women. Like her car, Robin's life had been marked by an illness. She was not contagious. The mark was not to ward off healthy people. It was a mark of courage, of sympathy, and of support. It meant that her identity had changed. She was a different person from the last time I saw her. Robin was a certified victim of breast cancer. Whether she would be a survivor remained to be seen.

WHY EVERYTHING IS PINK

Pink means breast cancer. More than that, the color is inextricably tied to cure, both through the subconscious association between "Find a cure!" logos and pink ribbons and through funneling money raised in those campaigns to cure-based research. While these pink products produce millions of dollars every year, few consumers question where that money is going. At the same time, attaching a pink ribbon to a product increases its value by making any company using it seem more philanthropic.

Breast cancer campaigns have depended on and reinforced the cultural cache of the pink ribbon—the symbol of breast cancer throughout the United States and now in other countries (Fernandez 1998; Moffett 2003). Sandy Fernandez, a writer for *MAMM* magazine, describes the way that the pink ribbon was created: "Sixty-eight-year-old Charlotte Haley began making peach ribbons after her daughter, sister and grandmother had breast cancer." She attached the ribbons to postcards that she sent out by the hundreds. Haley wrote on the card, "The National Cancer Institute annual budget is $1.8 billion, only 5 percent goes for cancer prevention. Help us wake up our legislators and America by wearing this ribbon" (Fernandez 1998).

That year, 1992, Alexandra Penney at *Self* magazine was in the midst of developing the second NBCAM campaign. The campaign had been a hit the prior year, but she wanted to make it better. Haley had been writing letters, sending her postcard to as many people as her personal budget would allow. The peach ribbon was gaining popularity. Penney heard about it and approached Haley, who was interested in using it. But Haley refused because she felt that *Self* and Estée Lauder, the makeup company working with *Self*, were too commercial. The two companies went to their lawyers, asking if they could use the ribbon without Haley's permission. Lawyers told them that there might be legal problems with that, so they should change the color. The two companies ran a series of focus groups asking women what color most reminded them of femininity, comfort, and support. Based on the results, Estée Lauder chose pink. Penney incorporated the ribbon into that month's advertising about breast exams and breast cancer awareness. The rest is history.

That year, Estée Lauder gave out 1.5 million pink ribbons and collected 200,000 pink ribbon petitions that were sent to Congress asking for more research funding. And the funding began to grow. "Between 1991 and 1996, federal funding for breast cancer research increased nearly fourfold to over $550 million," Fernandez (1998) reports. This funding was massively augmented by individual donations and new foundations dedicated to the disease, like Estée Lauder's Breast Cancer Research Foundation, the Komen Foundation, the Avon Foundation, and others. In 1996, the *New York Times Magazine* called breast cancer "this year's hot charity." Now, the pink ribbon awareness T-shirt sells at Wal-Mart for $5.86, Vendio sells twelve beaded pink ribbon key chains for $11.99, and Song-Delta Airlines has a white plane with a pink ribbon painted around it. According to sociologist Emily Kolker (2004), the pink ribbon campaign has successfully created "a deeper sense of public concern about breast cancer" (831). Women with the disease and their allies have used this symbol as a way to express support and community. At runs and walks, it is blown up on a large scale to unite the participants, while on a day-to-day basis, individuals wear pins and T-shirts that underline their membership in a particular group.

The pink ribbon is a symbol that mediates two sets of interests—the financially powerful who use it to drive consumption and those affected by breast cancer who wish to alleviate suffering, be that emotional or physical. It is a convenient meeting of the minds. The needs of two parties converge. One pursues financial profits, and the other, in our consumer society, soothes itself by buying things. As a symbol, it resolves a dichotomy in American illness, that is, the need to spend and the need to support. On a conceptual level, it "directly concerns the dramatic interplay and interaction of the opposing forces in the dualistic world of manifestation, their conflicting but also complementary and compensating characteristics" (Cirlot 1971, 8). The pink ribbon allows us to spend, something we are consistently compelled to do in America, rather than grieve. But it often seems that this symbol denies the devastation of the disease: families torn apart by medical costs, children scarred by the loss of their mothers, and women lost. The pink ribbon's use to support finding a cure precludes interest in prevention, which would be a way to honor the suffering of so many women. This is despite the intention of the ribbon's original creator.

WALKING, RACING, SHOPPING

As NBCAM has become an accepted period of commemoration, diverse fund-raisers have crossed the nation. The typical dinner or banquet has been overrun with exercise events. Over the years, these events have reached beyond the month of October and are now held year-round. They can also be found all over the country, mostly in major cities. Their size varies with location, ranging from a few hundred to tens of thousands of participants. Their purposes are often in the spirit of "empowering women (and men!), ensuring quality care for all, and energizing science," like the Susan G. Komen Foundation Race for the Cure Three-Day Walk (Komen 2007a). Like-minded folks gather together. There is a powerful camaraderie built while tears are shed and friends remembered.

Collecting documents and doing background research on breast cancer activism, I scanned files of photographs portraying walkers and magazine articles about the funds raised. Women in bright pink T-shirts smiled, hugging one another. Just looking at the photos, they all seemed so happy. For the most part, these rallies maintained a positive note, recognizing the losses endured while focusing on overcoming. But everything else I had been learning about breast cancer seemed so grim. I was sure that the camaraderie was heartfelt. I was also reading critiques of these marches. Many claimed that organizers were trying to avoid upsetting people in a way that might alienate them from the cause.

Eventually, I began to attend these events. Their popularity, vendors, and attendance shocked and amazed me—hundreds of thousands of people, usually wearing pink, raising money and building solidarity around an illness taking the lives of so many women. Going to any event made me cry—the dedication of the participants, the pain they had endured, and the wishes they had to alleviate suffering. In 2005, I set off for the ACS's Making Strides Against Breast Cancer. Cafés on Fifth Avenue and Lexington near the 72nd Street entrance to Central Park on Manhattan's East Side were jammed with people in pink T-shirts. They wore sweatpants and tennis shoes and chatted around coffee and danishes. Inside the park, pink became even more prevalent, and the sound of a loudspeaker, an announcer, then a live band, was audible as I approached.

The day was crisp and beautiful. A clear sky shone on the groups of mainly female walkers of every description. An African American mother and her sister pushed a stroller with an eight-year-old girl traipsing behind. A group of women clumped tightly together hustled into a tent, speaking Spanish rapidly and laughing high-pitched giggles. A few men were interspersed with the women. They were all older, seemingly serious, or maybe just feeling out of place.

The walk had started early that morning, around 8:30. Participants followed a black concrete trail from the main stage, where performers led aerobics and sang gospel music, through the park, then back to an adjacent area where they could pick up bottled water and nuts or trail mix. Some women wore bright pink feathered boas, while others carried pom-poms. Clowns circulated through the crowd, smiling and throwing kisses.

Making Strides has been growing since its initiation in 1993. The year 2005 saw an immense financial success, raising $32 million. The ACS has invested $246 million in cancer research since 1972 when President Nixon initiated the war on cancer. The walks are important to keeping the research going. As a walker, I wanted to know what was being done with the money. At the ACS walk, the emcee of the event announced that ACS officials direct all the money to research, treatment, and support, an agenda approved by the ACS board. Details were fuzzy. Even in the press packet, full of references to hotlines, the efficacy of mammography, and a pink ribbon, no information was being distributed about what the ACS does with the funds. Yet hundreds of thousands of people participate each year. I began to wonder what most walkers knew about where their money was going.

The next event I attended was an ACS walk in Boston. There, I decided to find out. Streams of women, gaggles of children, and a few men wove their way along the Charles River. The cold winter wind whipped up short, choppy waves that bit the late-blooming grasses at sidewalk's edge. The main stage area was full of walkers, informational booths, and a mammography van. Like the New York event, by early morning thousands of people were getting ready to make the short walk, sponsored by friends.

I had brought my video camera in order to capture how most of the public engages with breast cancer, something that would be important for the film I was making. It was easy to talk to people from behind the camera. The emcee had announced that Discovery Health Channel was making a film about breast cancer, so people were ready to talk with the camera rolling. I approached a group of six women wearing long-sleeve white T-shirts with pink lettering on the back, "Judy's team."

"Hi, there," I said as they turned around and smiled at me, seeing the camera hanging down by my side. "Can I ask you some questions?" "Sure," several of them replied. I asked who they were walking for. Each replied differently: a mother, a sister, a friend Judy. Was this their first time? Yes, second or fifth. How much money were they raising? About $4,000. What would the money be used for? Breast cancer research. What kind? The smiles turned to blank expressions. I looked from one member of the group to the next. "We are not sure," was the final answer. "The American Cancer Society will decide."

I said good-bye and wished them well on their walk. Other groups stood talking in the grassy area surrounding the registration booth. A couple of teenagers stood apart from a larger group of twenty or so people wearing bright orange T-shirts. I asked them about their experience with the walk. This was the third year for this team. So far, they had raised $20,000. Again, they were not sure where the money was going. Other groups were the same. Some wore team shirts, and others wore sweatpants or jeans. Some made this an annual event. Others were coming for the first time. These walkers were pulling in large sums of money. Few knew where the money was going. I didn't know either. I decided to find out.

WHERE DOES THE MONEY GO?

Estimating the total amount of dollars circulating throughout the breast cancer industry is difficult, especially considering the vast number of cancer centers, radiation centers, breast health centers, hospital care units, surgical procedures, and hormonal treatment regimens. Twelve to sixteen billion is one estimate (Ehrenreich 2001) of how much we spend on breast cancer annually. And this number does not include many of the research dollars used to address it. If accurate, that would mean that the disease and its affiliated costs are more than 10 percent of the American gross domestic product.

Philanthropic efforts represent one part of this estimation. Large sums of money are raised at breast cancer walks, from related product sales and other cause-marketing campaigns, so much that the Komen Foundation has committed to dedicating $1 billion to the disease in the next decade. Calculating how much is raised annually in total is difficult if not impossible. With all the products and events dedicated to breast cancer, the cause is too large and diffuse to decipher, even more so for figuring out what the money is used for. Many organizations do not clarify the destination of most donations.

One group of activists that calls itself Follow the Money, led by Karen Miller of the Huntington Breast Cancer Action Coalition on Long Island; the New York State Breast Cancer Network; the Women's Cancer Resource Center in Minnesota; Barbara Brenner, director of Breast Cancer Action; Deb Forter of the Massachusetts Breast Cancer Coalition; and other organizations have tried to analyze the numbers and make the administrators of walk events accountable to those who bring in the dollars. They first targeted the Avon Foundation. It is one of the largest breast cancer foundations in the country, and at the same time, the Avon Corporation makes millions of dollars selling products to women. The group argued that raising money for breast cancer could be a marketing ploy on the part of the corporation. With this reasoning, they set out to make sure that the money raised was going somewhere beneficial to women.

Avon's walk is serious compared to most others. It takes up to a whole weekend, with one group of walkers picking the twenty-six-mile marathon length. The more hardy participants endure a marathon and a half. The Crusade for the Cure was first created in the United Kingdom in 1992, then launched in the United States in 1993. Its name was changed to the Breast Cancer Walk in 2002. As of 2002, fund-raising activities were already held in fifty countries. The total raised from outside the United States was $235,000. Ten years into the walks, 600 programs have been sponsored worldwide, 114 of these in the United States (see table 2.2).

A letter from Susan Heaney, director of public relations, to Breast Cancer Action, the Massachusetts Breast Cancer Coalition, and a few other organizations details Avon's activities. These projects have been run through the Avon Foundation, but the Avon Corporation foots a lot of the bill. Each year it spends more than $20 million on breast cancer. "Taken individually or as a

Table 2.2. Money Raised in Breast Cancer Events

Event (2004)	Money Raised
Avon's Breast Cancer Crusade	$6,514,016
Avon Public Awareness	$5,389,507
American Cancer Society Walks	$32,000,000
Susan G. Komen Foundation Race for the Cure	$96,913,909

whole," Heaney wrote, "we believe that Avon is among the very best corporate leaders in the world in support of a charitable cause."

The letter from Heaney was in response to criticisms from the campaign. Breast Cancer Action, in particular, had been leafleting with a brochure that read, "Think twice before you do the Avon 3-Day Walk!" The foldout read that more than a third of the money raised for Avon would not go to breast cancer programs and that the company refused to guarantee that women who lived in the areas where funds were raised could play a role in deciding how those funds would be used. Instead, a thirty-person panel from across the country administered the funds. Women from organizations in the Follow the Money Coalition had written letters arguing against Avon and demanding that local organizations be allowed to help decide where the money would go.

The fall of 2001 brought the two sides together in the Avon boardroom in New York City to discuss the issue. The Follow the Money Coalition had come to meet with four Avon officials. Questions were mounting. It was unclear how much was going back to research, support, and other areas that fund-raisers were claiming to be the purpose of the events. The group wanted these questions answered and wanted to make sure that each town where money was raised received some of the proceeds.

Criticizing breast cancer efforts was a sensitive prospect. Women had struggled for years just to get the public to pay attention to the illness. A huge amount of courage and dedication had been necessary for Happy Rockefeller and Betty Ford to go public with their experiences. These walks and runs were a part of the legacy begun by those individual women. Tens of thousands of survivors participate in them each year, remembering loved ones and reaching out to others. The Follow the Money Coalition did not want to defame these efforts but rather wanted to make the companies managing the money more accountable. It was a delicate situation.

Brenner wrote in a newsletter, "If you are one of the thousands of people who have put considerable energy into efforts like the Avon 3-Day, know that we cherish and applaud your commitment and encourage you to join us in our continuing efforts to create the changes necessary to end the breast cancer epidemic." But in another newsletter, a real concern about the way that participants think about the walk emerged. Ellen Leopold, a member of Breast Cancer Action, wrote that "women are once again donating their time, energy, and money, *no questions asked*."

Avon offices are in the midst of Manhattan, between 54th and 55th streets on Sixth Avenue. The Follow the Money Coalition met there with Avon. Kathleen Walas, president of the vast and financially powerful Avon Products Foundation, was there to answer concerns. Tom Sarakatsannis, the only man in the room, was a member of the foundation's board. Susan Heaney, the public relations vice president for the foundation, was there to supervise. Mendocino County was one example that Barbara raised. That county had some of the highest rates of breast cancer in California. The Northern California Avon Walk had drawn more than $15,000 from Mendocino. At the same time, 70 percent of local cancer support center funds were being raised from community donations. Its budget was $140,000. The locals needed as much money as they could get their hands on for breast cancer, but thousands of dollars were going to Avon rather than back to the community where cancer rates were high.

In addition, they raised a different point: Avon was taking money out of the earnings of the walks and using it to pay for advertising, promoting, and organizing. Thirty-five percent of the money raised went to Pallotta Team-Works, the company that administered the walks for Avon. Susan and Kathleen were conciliatory. They knew that the activists represented constituents all over the United States and had the ability to influence public opinion. While a lot of people did not know what happened behind the scenes at the Avon Products Foundation, the Follow the Money Coalition could inform them. They promised to look into it, make changes, and figure out how to streamline the walks.

Other concerned activists were already writing in. "As someone who works in the nonprofit field and shares your commitment to ending breast cancer, I appreciate Avon's commitment to this devastating disease," wrote Sue Newman from her home in Martinez, California. "I would however like to express some of my concerns." Her letter continued, "I'm sure you realize that anything over 30 percent going to administrative costs in a fund-raising event is considered mismanagement of good donor dollars. Avon would be able to give more money to organizations doing the type of work that is needed and would gain a better reputation as a company that takes the time and effort to support programs making a real difference."

The letter had been directed to Kathleen Walas and Andrea Jung. Three days later, they sent a response. "Each year, Avon Products, Inc. spends in excess of $20,000,000 on the breast cancer cause to cover its widespread philanthropic activities around the world," Susan Heaney wrote. "Avon has provided corporate-salaried staff support, on-site personnel at the events, and Avon products for nearly every participant (totaling $1,000,000 annually). Financial information about the Walks is disclosed on every donor form, on our websites, and in printed materials about the events."

The activists read the response as "Forget it. We are doing a good job, and that's what we are going to keep on doing." Brenner decided to take public action. Breast Cancer Action bought a *New York Times* ad; a whole page cost $75,000. The ad ran with the headline "Who's Really Cleaning Up Here?" A

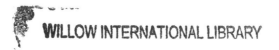

large red vacuum cleaner moved along a smooth, dark floor. Eureka donates one dollar for every vacuum in the Clean for the Cure promotion. American Express gives one penny for every transaction in its Charge for the Cure campaign. Next to these facts, the vacuum looked ridiculous, not like a benefit to charity but like a way to reinforce stereotypes about women. These new ads by Breast Cancer Action provided a new look at these fund-raising and advertising campaigns. They are not just about the disease but could also be looked at as promotional advertising for the companies running them (File and Prince 2004). More vacuum cleaners get sold, more Avon products get bought, and more money gets charged on American Express cards. Those companies make more profits. They benefit from the philanthropic cause attached to their names (Polonsky and Wood 2001).

At the next Avon annual shareholder meeting, Jung, Avon's chief executive officer (CEO), was perfectly manicured and suited. She was a feminine businesswoman, the ideal representative of Avon. She stood in front of the shareholders describing new business developments and announced that year as the last for the Avon Three-Day Walks. Instead, Avon would invest in new fund-raising vehicles. Because of the pushing and negotiating of the Follow the Money Coalition, Avon changed its practices.

Many other walks have opaque practices. Few participants question whose hands the money ends up in and what the motivation is for each organization to hold its walk. Questioning philanthropy is taboo. Yet many of the companies increasing sales from cause marketing already make more than enough. The largest financial gains go to the CEOs of large companies. For example, the CEO of the ACS makes over $900,000 annually (ACS 2005). Not far behind are the CEOs of the Breast Cancer Research Foundation, founded by Estée Lauder, who make $444,000 (Estée Lauder Companies 2005). Komen CEOs make almost half, around $222,000 (Komen Foundation 2006). (See figure 2.1). Meanwhile, the market for their products continues to expand, and women continue to get sick with breast cancer.

The morning of the surgery, the alarm went off at 4:15, August 31, 2004. The sky was lit only by a half moon that hung bright white over a horizon of buttermilk clouds. Sheaves of sea grass next to the driveway shifted and brushed against one another, hushing the ocean tides nearby. The kitchen was bright with fluorescent light. Only Tori and Little Eddy were awake, sitting with their grandfather next to the shiny gray and black marbletop island in the middle of the room. Little Eddy stared at a set of blue flippers with green trim he had just been given. Tori tried new ringtones on her cell phone, each chirping clip brighter and cheerier than the last.

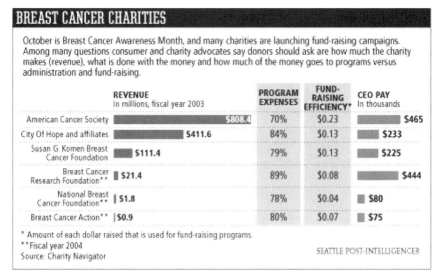

Figure 2.1. Disbursement of Breast Cancer Charity Revenue

Robin wore a white tank top and jeans with colored stitching. She poured coffee from a silver carafe into two Styrofoam cups, then leaned against the counter to watch the kids. She sipped the coffee with a half smile on her face, eyes unfocused, watching something in her own mind. She had decided to have both breasts removed. The type of cancer the doctors found in her left breast was almost guaranteed to eventually invade her right. Removing that breast was a prophylactic measure. Removing the left was immediately necessary.

Robin's father had driven two hours from Connecticut in his white Mercedes to help take care of the kids. The kitchen was bright and seemingly carefree. Robin tried to organize the room, knowing that when she was strong enough to do that again, it would be a mess. "All right, let's do this," Robin said almost to herself as she wiped down the countertop. Her hair was down and draped almost white blond across her shoulders, hiding her face as she scrubbed the surface. Eddy was rushing from upstairs to downstairs, then to the basement and back to the kitchen, busy with a multitude of tasks.

"We should get going," Eddy said, stopping to lean over little Eddy and his new flippers. Robin agreed and they began their good-byes. There was nothing to collect or organize. The small black duffel bag containing the things she might need to stay in the hospital for a few days was already in the car. The hospital had all her records. Eddy went to warm up the car.

"Okay, Dad, you all set? We're gonna go," Robin said to her dad.

"Fine, fine. Everything is fine," he replied. She kissed him and then the kids together.

"I love you," Robin called backward into the house as she stepped out of the front door. The ocean breeze was rife with sea life. It swept its way into the house as she shut the door behind her and walked briskly to the pearl white SUV. Eddy had already started it and was waiting in the driveway for her. Robin walked out, empty-handed, into the dark morning.

The drive to the hospital was short. The sun had not yet risen. They parked the car in the lot, which was surprisingly full, and went through the sliding glass doors into the surgery sector. I followed them, feeling like I did not belong.

Chapter Three

Where We Might Go

Breast cancer would hardly be the darling of corporate America if its complexion changed from pink to green.

—Barbara Ehrenreich

The color had left her cheeks. Her arms hung motionless off the side of the bed. All four limbs had fallen straight, perfectly relaxed like a child sleeping. Her mane was tucked into an antiseptic blue hair cap keeping it off her nude body. Two middle-aged nurses picked her up. Two young men came rushing in to help. They expertly avoided gliding in slippery surgical footies. The four of them lifted her comatose figure from the bed to the table.

The nurses began to work. Her body was mapped onto the table, arms tied with wristbands, legs held down with a heavy black rubber belt, feet wrapped in mechanical white socks that massaged blood through her legs. Layers of material were swathed one after the other over her exposed body, first a film of corrugated plastic, then a white cotton cloth followed by a blue one. A drape was hung between two poles at the head of the bed. Her head popped off the top of her torso like a cork, no longer visible to us.

Her breasts ascended from the mountain of fabric colored like an open sky. Spotlights beamed on them. The tan lines that started on her collarbones continued over her breasts. They were bone white. I felt cold. I imagined she was too. None of the nurses appeared embarrassed by this brash nakedness. I had never been attached to my breasts. I had often wondered about the American obsession with them. Size, shape, nipple color—it all seemed so irrelevant.

My mind wanted to focus elsewhere to evade the disturbing scene. It reverted to the past.

"Hey! You made it," Robin had said to me as I arrived at her house the first time we met. Her daughter was shy and only looked at me. Robin gave me a hug. "You're so cute. Look at you."

I looked at her. She was barely ten years older than I. We crossed the short driveway and undersized lawn into the house. After passing through the kitchen, we met the rest of the family in the back. Robin's six-year-old son swam in a modest kidney-shaped pool. Her teenage daughter stood at the edge of the deck with a friend. Robin's husband sat at the glass table pecking it with his fingertips and talking on the phone. He was different than he had sounded on voice mail. His voice had been rough and nasal, his manner businesslike and curt. In person, his soft belly and floral shorts made him less daunting, somehow more human. He was dark and Italian, a lover of his family.

Eddy had been forced to leave the pre-op room before the surgeons came. I stayed with Robin. I wasn't even family. He was her lifeblood. He would return in eight hours after the surgery was over. In the meantime, he would stop at the drugstore for lozenges, help Robin's mother to use the bathroom, drop the kids off, and briefly fall asleep on the couch at home. Robin and I talked, but her throat was dry from the mouthwash beginning to take effect. I had to fill the gap of her usually quick tongue and constant words. But the tightness in my chest and lightness in my head distracted me.

First the plastic surgeon came in. Lloyd and Robin had known each other since high school. Robin couldn't remember if they had ever made out. She stood in front of him bare chested with a dotted gown wrapped around her waist. He removed a black marker from his pocket and drew on her torso, front and back, pulling at her flesh, measuring, estimating, and planning. The general surgeon came in a few minutes later. Lloyd had been wearing a suit. This man was already in scrubs. He did not smile and made no comforting gestures. The nurses listened to his directions. He left. They stayed and administered to Robin—forms, drugs, and questions. Then they wheeled her away. The hallway was dim, a catacomb of rooms, passageways, and offices, each floor repeating the one before. I would never be able to find my way back.

Above the drape the anesthesiologist inserted a tube into Robin's throat. A face mask of drugs had lulled her, and sleep was imminent, but she coughed with reproach as the shaft was delivered into her trachea. My mouth filled with the heat of nausea and tears. The fleshy woman murmured soft words to Robin. She would remember none of this later and would ask me to describe it. I would avoid her questions. The surgeons came in holding wet, freshly washed hands in the air. Nurses wrapped them in gowns, and they immediately began demanding tools in high, sharp voices.

Lloyd drew on her chest, then cut into flesh in a circular line around the nipple, then straight down opening the breast below it. I have yet to register the impact the first cut made on my psyche. It was not like watching a movie. But it was far from real. Blood began to seep through miniscule fault lines formulated by precise instruments. It dripped over the black trails of a master plan. I stepped away as I had been instructed to do if faintness approached. I was sure blackness would come, but it didn't. Piercing overhead lights insistently reminded me of where I was and that there was no easy escape. I had brought this on myself, documenting a double mastectomy as a part of the film. I had not only known what I was getting into but also asked for it. There had been no real way to prepare for it.

"If the incision is made correctly," said Lloyd, narrating the surgery, "the patient shouldn't bleed a great deal." He had already put staples in to mark the bottom of the breast. That had been their first invasion into her body. It was childish and simplistically odd for such a complicated surgery. Pulling apart the skin they had separated with the first cut, the surgeons pulled the dripping red flesh of the breast out, then did away with it, and moved on to the next breast. After each one was empty of possibly carcinogenic flesh, they stapled it closed and flat to her chest. They were then done with what they called the simple mastectomy.

That day, both breasts would be removed, and latissimus tissue would be inserted in their place. Under the tissue taken from her back and pulled through into her chest, plastic bulbs would be inserted. Over the weeks to come, these tissue expanders would slowly be filled with saline, stretching the breasts back to their original size or larger. In a year, Robin would have two new breasts to replace the cancerous ones. Once the summer rolled around again, she would be ready to go back to the beach. Almost no sign would be left of today's seemingly endless procedure. Robin had told me all this. I hoped she was right. That this would be the end of it. No more worries, no more mammograms.

It had taken the general surgeon less than two hours. Now the plastic surgeon stepped in. His eyes were blank, trained on the skin in front of him. Many women with breast cancer would not have had this second part of the surgery. Sutures would have completed the operation, leaving a level chest and horizontal scars.

"Robin had breast implants put in seven years ago," said Lloyd. "We'll add new ones eventually, once she has healed from this operation."

"Have you ever been in an operating room before?" he asked.

"Only as a patient," I replied.

His eyebrows rose fleetingly, but he did not look at me.

Now nurses laid Robin on her stomach, and Lloyd drew an oblong circular form on the left side of her back with the same thick, black ink. Lamps pulled close to the table shone on the top of his head, making his white surgical bonnet radiate light. He was angelic and dangerous, God-like and mortal. More cuts were made on her back. The smell of burning flesh made me gag. Lloyd described his work to me as he gently tugged and separated the muscles. His voice came down a tunnel to my ears. There was no more human form there on the table. Only blazing red and the fall orange of iodine floating in a sea of blue. The colors merged and separated, playing against one another in combat. My eyes readjusted. I focused.

Hours passed. I watched and listened.

Robin's consciousness returned quickly. She blubbered unintelligible words, sounds, something about water and nausea. The room that had been sealed shut with surgical secrecy and cleanliness was now exposed. Both doors had been flung open, and doctors, nurses, and administrators walked by, sometimes glancing in. The last shift of nurses was performing a thorough cleaning, clear plastic bags full of blue, red, and white unidentifiable objects being carried out. Heart-shaped buckets of dirty water were dumped. Soiled instruments were gathered together and counted once, then twice, then a third time to make sure that nothing had been lost or left inside Robin's body.

The recovery room was full of patients, most of them old and pale. Each bed was separated from the next by a flimsy sheet mostly pulled back by a hassled nurse taking care of too many patients, rushing from one bed to the next.

"Wake up, Jack!" said Robin's nurse. His eyes popped open. "You need to take a deep breath. Come on." Robin's neighbor was old and peaceful when not being called to attention by the nurse.

She looked at me, seeming to know who I was. In my glasses and blue uniform, surgical cap and face mask pulled down past my chin, I looked like a doctor. She knew I wasn't.

"How long was the surgery?" she asked.

"Eight hours, I think."

"You were in there the whole time?"

"I took a lunch break."

Robin cried out in pain. She had become magical to me, like she had passed through something impossible, inhuman, that made her otherworldly. I stood frozen several feet from her bed.

"Could you feed her these ice chips?" the nurse asked.

"Sure," I replied because there was no other answer. I took the white paper cup and spoon and shuffled to the bedside. Robin squirmed and turned to look up at me, opening her eyes only for an instant. Her thumb pressed down on the white button that would deliver pain medication. She turned away and rested. I looked at her gown with tiny teddy bears dancing across folds of twisted cloth. Her pale hand clutched and pulled at it, and her knuckles were white. I could only remember the whiteness of her breasts.

I walked down the hall to the changing room where I threw away my adopted scrubs and my temporary identity with it. The bin of dirty surgical gear overflowed onto the floor and across the room, and footies were littered in every corner. I emerged from the locker room and headed down the hallway back to the recovery room, stopping on my way to glance out the window, remembering that there was a world outside where the sun was beginning to warm as the afternoon wore on and where the parking lot was already beginning to empty. Eddy's unwieldy SUV was parked among the other cars, seemingly undetailed squares of black, silver, and green from the fifth-floor window.

I turned and walked on, anticipating meeting him with feigned cheerfulness in the post-op room. As I turned down the hallway, I saw his back. He sat hunched over Robin, gently swaying. He was crying.

TWO NEW WAVES OF ACTIVISM

Many decades have passed since science was conceived of as developing in a vacuum—the money that funds it, the agencies that issue requests for proposals, and the public that demands that the study of new illnesses guide research and, in some people's words, form "bandwagons" of research topics and approaches almost impossible to dismantle. Breast cancer research is no different. Government agencies, followed by large pharmaceutical companies, initiated the breast cancer research agenda. Eventually, activists joined the struggle and tried to reshape it. These groups grew over the years but not on an even playing field. And their agendas were far from the same. The second wave of activists publicized mammography as prevention, got services like prostheses and transportation to treatment for women, and generated awareness about breast cancer among the general public (Gardner 2006).

A third wave of activism gained prominence in the 1990s and are the best-known breast cancer activists today. They made demands for women with the disease and to redirect the bandwagons or at least get on board. They wanted to be involved in policymaking and represented on scientific review panels for government-funded research. This would give women with breast cancer some voice in research without being too radical.

A fourth and most recent wave of breast cancer activism then emerged mainly on Long Island, in Massachusetts, and in San Francisco with sister organizations popping up around the globe. In these hot spots of breast cancer activism, women argued that more of the same was simply not enough. In some cases, these activists were bold enough to claim that advocacy groups, government, and especially the corporations were doing it all wrong. They criticized the traditional research trajectory based on money from big business. They wanted to know what was driving breast cancer rate increases, what was causing the loss of years of women's lives. Soon enough, these women would initiate an entirely new research agenda, make regulations for chemicals tighter, and change the public face of breast cancer.

This controversial activism has flown in the face of most awareness raising. The research they have instigated about what causes breast cancer is scientifically challenging. New research methods and tools have to be developed to answer the complex questions posed by nonscientists free from norms of professional training (Brown et al. 2006). But activists do not base the need for this research only on a gut feeling. There are data, years long and bridging many scientific fields, that show diverse causes of the disease. Gasoline additives, paints, food packaging, and many other products have been linked to breast cancer (Rudel et al. 2007).

Mainstream breast cancer researchers have often viewed these studies as spurious and insignificant, a set of data not big enough to be considered seriously. In the world of Thomas Kuhn (1962), one of the world's most famous historians of science, these studies are actually a researcher's misstep away from "normal science," or the puzzles and questions that conform to mainstream scientific research. Only over a period of time when more and more of these missteps aggregate can they actually overturn traditional scientific bandwagons. Such a "paradigm shift" has the potential to create a crisis in science and revolutionize its outcomes. But changing the focus of breast cancer research from detection, treatment, and cure would be more than a scientific revolution. It would mean changing policy and production practices.

The scientists moving in the direction of disease causation research have faced a constant storm. Other scientists have largely ignored this work or, worse yet, berated its authors. The biggest newspapers have called research on environmental links methodologically unsound and based on superstition. Possibly even more difficult than this backlash is the entrenched research approach based in a lab that ignores factors outside an individual's body. This scientific method became the basis of modern medicine around the turn of the twentieth century when germ theory took shape and when polluting industrial companies used it to shirk responsibility for their impact on public health (Tesh 1988). Over the years, companies have used this as a way to sidestep their responsibility for disease causation. Although science seems objective, sociologist Joan Busfield (2007) argues that "an important source of its [the pharmaceutical industry's] power is in the control it exerts over the scientific fact making" (423). By focusing on the transmission of germs or individual risk factors, they drive public concern about it, keeping attention away from exposures that they might have caused.

Geoffrey Rose (1992), a scientist famous for radical prevention measures for coronary artery disease, best explained why a focus on the illness of individuals instead of whole groups or communities does not work. He used drunk driving as an example. "If a small amount of alcohol slightly impairs a driver's judgment, then the large number of drivers who have had one or two drinks would collectively incur a large excess of accidents, even though none of them individually had an obvious problem" (86), he explained.

This principle has been broadly applied to many other social and illness conditions. The link between toxins and breast cancer is the same. If one individual inhales chlorine when cleaning her bathroom and eats pesticides at the dinner table, over years they add up. However, because there are so many diverse sources, their link to cancer may not be apparent. Toxins add up in individuals and in entire populations. However, as Rose (1992) continued, "current policy assumes that this is not the case" (82). In other words, most research and policy treats the individual as an isolated case. This trend is now shifting toward an even more minute level, to genetics, drawing farther away from the environmental factors that flip genetic switches. A vastly disproportionate amount of funding is funneled into these topics while work directed at public health and environmental exposures has been marginalized. Economic reasons for this research trajectory abound. Most important, if the locus of disease causation is put in an individual's hands, responsibility for prevention falls away from polluters that could have caused it. Complicit government institutions therefore avoid fighting powerful and entrenched corporate actors, some of whom fund their election campaigns. Such politics are masked by a thin veil of medical and scientific neutrality, focusing solely on treatments that are seemingly unobjectionable, that is, until you look under the surface.

ESTABLISHING THE BREAST CANCER AGENDA

The vast majority of the research stimulated by Nixon's 1972 call to battle a "war" against cancer has used a biomedical approach. Elliot Mishler (1981) describes it as the unquestioned conceptual model on which medical thinking is based. A graying, wizened Harvard professor of psychiatry, Mishler has spent years analyzing the framework of medicine. As he describes it, the biomedical model's key assumptions are that there is a specific etiology, or cause, and that medicine is value free. This implies that there are no political economic or cultural factors driving treatment of disease. It puts most stock in individual-level risk factors for breast cancer like genetics and lifestyle. For example, researchers looking at causes of breast cancer have studied the potential increase in risk due to giving birth for the first time later in life, alcohol consumption, diet and exercise, genetic makeup, and other risk factors that operate at the individual level. This is the biggest research bandwagon. Most are on board. Despite the assumed neutrality of the biomedical model, there are political and scientific reasons that researchers use it.

Sheldon Krimsky, a professor at Tufts University who researches government spending on research and regulation, explained how we reached this state of matters. "In the 1960s, a number of government officials made the decision that it would be more economically beneficial to cure cancer than to prevent it" (personal communication, 2006). These officials knew that cancer rates were rising and that they were probably linked to the increasing number of chemicals being produced in industrial processes. Rather than slowing this usage down, they allowed more and more to be brought to market and instead started research campaigns to deal with chemical outcomes—cancer. Over the years, the government's agenda has been played out while more and more people have suffered the ravages of cancer.

LARGE PHARMACEUTICAL COMPANIES AND THE BASICS OF BREAST CANCER

American politeness, reflected in hesitancy to discuss the intimate details of illness, has hidden the rise and power of the pharmaceutical industry. Probably the majority of your friends and family are on some sort of prescribed drug, and, in fact, the National Health Service of England issues 12.5 prescriptions per person (Busfield 2007). While this is exceedingly normal to us now, it has not always been this way. The pharmaceutical industry has grown rapidly since the world wars. The ending of these wars and the growth of large pharmaceutical companies is no coincidence. The massive funds and technologies invested in chemical proliferation for warfare suddenly lost their significance when Hitler's regime was dismantled and guns were laid to rest (Daniel 2006). New markets emerged to use these chemicals. Mass marketing and consumption of pharmaceuticals and industrial chemicals were the result, the former growing out of the latter (Nelson 1999).

Some argue that breast cancer sits at the intersection of these two industries—the same companies that once produced industrial chemicals now make pharmaceuticals. This is not scientific coincidence; the skills to make these products and run such companies overlap. These pharmaceutical companies are massive, and the most profitable industry in America (Center for Policy Alternatives 2000) (see table 3.1). One of the most lucrative companies in this position has been AstraZeneca, the very same company that owns the copyright to National Breast Cancer Awareness Month. AstraZeneca originated in the form of Imperial Chemical Industries (ICI). At first, ICI developed and marketed a vast assortment of products—adhesives, specialty synthetic polymers, electronic and engineering materials, explosives, soda ash, rubber chemicals, sulfur-related products, fibers, natural and synthetic lubricants, and eventually personal care products and food ingredients (Taylor and Sudnick 1984). It invented an acrylic plastic called Perspex in 1932 for lighting, Plexiglas, and other products. With DuPont, Dulux paints were also created and used widely in homes and businesses.

By the 1940s, ICI had already moved into the pharmaceutical sector. That decade, it began manufacturing an antimalarial, paludrine, still commonly taken by travelers more than sixty years later. The year 1950 marked the production of halothane, an inhaled anesthetic agent often used in veterinarian surgery or for humans in developing nations, after it was judged to be too toxic for human subjects in Europe. Often, toxic substances find a home in developing nations because of lax regulations, while those same substances are discontinued in

Table 3.1.   Select Breast Cancer Drugs—Usage and Profits

Drug	Usage	Company	2006 Profits
Abraxane	Chemotherapy	Abraxis Bioscience	$174.9 million
Aredia	Adjuvant	Novartis	* (in litigation
Arimidex	Post-surgery	AstraZeneca	$1.5 billion
Ellence	Chemotherapy	Pfizer	$320 million
Faslodex	Early stage treatment	AstraZeneca	$186 million
Femara		Novartis	$719 million
Herceptin	Adjuvant therapy, post-chemo	Roche	$3.9 billion
Taxotere	During chemo or after	Sanofi-Aventis Pharmaceuticals	$1.75 billion
Tamoxifen	Post-surgery treatment	AstraZeneca	$89 million
Taxol		Bristol Meyers-Squibb	$563 million
Xeloda	Adjuvant treatment	Roche	$971 million
Zoladex	Advanced breast cancer	AstraZeneca	$1 billion
Zometa	Cancer complications	Novartis	$696 million (in litigation)
			TOTAL *$11, 869 billion*

Note: Data for this table was compiled from 2006 annual reports from each company.
Information was unavailable for Adriamycin (Pfizer), Aromasin (Pfizer), Cytoxan (Bristol Meyers-Squibb), and Fareston (Shire Roberts).

richer nations. Halothane was followed in 1965 by a tranquilizer, Inderal, which soothes nervous system responses to stress.

In 1978, ICI copyrighted Tamoxifen, a breast cancer drug. Researchers invented this seeming miracle that would flow through the bloodstream and lock with the hormone receptors of breast cancer cells. This would stop estrogen, a catalyst of breast cancer growth, from linking with cancerous mammary cells, therefore slowing cancer recurrence. Later, researchers also guessed it could be used on women without the disease but with a family history in order to lower risk. By the early 1990s, Tamoxifen was on the market. Little did the makers realize that because of bad scientific guesses, administrative mishaps, and other contradictory products the company sold, Tamoxifen would become the most controversial breast cancer drug ever made and one of ICI's most publicized ventures (BBC News 1998; Food and Drug Adminstration [FDA] 1998; Rosser 2000).

At first, Tamoxifen seemed like a miracle drug. It reduced the chances of women who had breast cancer getting it again. In the early 1990s, the Breast Cancer Prevention Trial, partially funded by the National Cancer Institute, tested Tamoxifen on thousands of women. Then, based on initial evidence, doctors decided to start giving it to women with a family history of breast cancer who wanted to decrease their risk (Zones 2000). By the late 1990s, the drug was being perscribed commonly, yet it still did not have FDA approval. There was a loophole. Healthy women were being enrolled in a drug trial for Tamoxifen based on the evidence for sick women, including those defined "at risk" simply because they were over the age of sixty (Fisher 1997). Then patients, both healthy and sick, started reporting side effects: dizziness, memory loss, hot flashes, and liver tumors. Several women died of uterine cancer. The National Women's Health Network charged that tens of thousands of women had not been told about the risks. Government hearings brought their testimonies forward, and soon the drug trial ended. Tamoxifen prescriptions for sick women continued, but sales declined, and the company began to look for alternative drugs.

With AstraZeneca (and possibly many other corporations), there has been an overlap in production and consumption—the company has manufactured both carcinogenic chemicals and cancer treatments. ICI gave birth to AstraZeneca during its 1993 demerger of its Pharmaceuticals, Agrochemicals, and Specialties sectors. Zeneca's top productivity lines were agrochemicals, including Gramoxone, Fusilade, Touchdown, and Surpass, all herbicides; Karate, an insecticide; and Amistar, a fungicide. Total sales equal 5.5 billion British pounds. Zeneca then joined with Astra, a Swedish firm. Their specialties were a different line of pharmaceuticals and medical devices. Together, these two companies formed AstraZeneca. Some of the company's most popular products were in oncology, Zoladex, Casodex, Nolvadex, otherwise known as tamoxifen citrate, and Arimidex. These are some of the most popularly used breast cancer drugs in the world.

This overlap did not last long. In 1999, AstraZeneca demerged its pesticide production to focus more on pharmaceuticals (Ramirez and Tylecote 2002). The streamlining paid off. In 2003, Arimidex, a breast cancer treatment drug, made $519 million. That year, its sales climbed 46 percent, rising above the popularity of Tamoxifen. Faslodex made $77 million in sales, and Zoladex resulted in $869 million. Brent Vose, head of oncology for AstraZeneca in 2002, presented the rationale for continued investment in these drugs: the rising incidence of cancer, an aging population, and earlier diagnosis. His colleague's PowerPoint presentation detailed more specifically that the company has "a unique franchise in breast and prostate cancer" and that "the move into early disease represents an enormous expansion of the potential market" (Blackledge 2002). An increasing number of cases means more sales. Catching breast cancer earlier also means more people to treat. The reasoning for manufacturing certain drugs is at once practical and decidedly troubling. Data broken down into pie charts and graphs shows the massive numbers of disease victims who must be treated. It also reduces human suffering and death into a simple descriptive statistical profile, lines on a chart, representing a market demand waiting to be met.

ICI is one of many companies that in its initial years produced chemicals but quickly expanded to drug treatments—a decidedly lucrative market today. Lustful for profits, an exceedingly convenient surprise awaited these manufacturers: their second market grew out of the first. Industrial chemicals caused many illnesses for which pharmaceuticals are the treatment today. Some might say that pharmaceuticals are the cleanup crew for human destruction caused by man-made chemicals. Our massive exposure to chemicals causes cancers, brain disorders, nervous system malfunction, autism, skin rashes, respiratory problems—an endless number of illnesses. We use pharmaceuticals to treat them. For this reason, the chemical age was the precursor to what has become the pharmaceutical age. Strange bedfellows indeed.

TREATMENT FOR ROBIN

Following the operation, Robin had two months to regain enough strength before entering her first round of chemotherapy. Her body had not healed entirely, and the reconstruction was far from complete, but there was a need to start the process before any remnant cells could slip away to other parts of her body. The doctor's office was three miles from the house, close enough so that even if the chemo made her sick, she could still probably drive home on her own.

The office's squat brick building is protected from the road only by a parking lot and wooden sign advertising "Chemotherapy Services" with a telephone number in gold cursive lettering. The first time Robin arrived for treatment, it swung in the breeze. She parked the car and went in. The waiting room was unremarkable. Several patients of multiple ages sat reading magazines while a secretary behind a white counter typed at the computer. Robin checked in and sat down.

When her name was called, she went into a small, oblong entry room lined by counters. Just enough space was left for a small plastic chair and a stool. There, blood was taken and tested for white cell count. She sat waiting for the results and peeking through the next door where the treatment would actually take place. Eight sagging blue reclining chairs made out of rubber or leather were lined up with backs against the wall facing a row of cabinets. They were all full. It was like a factory assembly line with multiple patients moving out of one chair and another filling it anew, a constant stream of treatment.

Nurses buzzed around the room injecting chemicals into intravenous drips and leaning over to chat quietly with patients. Robin's nurse, Priscilla,[1] guided her into the room and to a chair next to a man in his seventies whose eyes peered toward a television in the other direction. A woman sat on her other side but did not stir as Robin settled in and pulled back her blond hair already growing dark at the roots. No hair dye was allowed during the chemo process. It might contribute to hair loss.

Priscilla hung a drip from a skinny metal pole next to Robin's chair and adjusted her bright blue sweatshirt. "Hold this back for me," she said brightly. "Like this?" Robin asked as she pulled the material away from below her collarbone. During her surgery, a port had been inserted there. Just under her skin was a piece of plastic that would make it easier for the nurse to find just where the needle should be inserted. Priscilla rubbed two fingers around the area, and Robin's skin slid and bulged as the plastic piece shifted underneath. She swept an alcohol-soaked cotton ball across the bulge and swiftly inserted the needle attached to a long, thin tube. "Okay?" she asked Robin. Robin nodded, her nose wrinkling and eyes glistening.

Priscilla went to the other end of the room where she sat down in front of a boxlike shelf in the wall guarded by a half sheet of Plexiglas. Behind it she pulled vials and needles, injecting several into the second drip that Robin would get in forty-five minutes. The countertop was spotlessly clean despite

---

[1]This name has been changed for anonymity.

how crowded it was. Lines of fat, squat glass bottles lined the shelves, organized by a colored band wrapped around their tops like little soldiers with funny hats. Priscilla finished mixing the next treatment and left the counter. Another nurse sat down. More patients came in.

Robin sat quietly, watching and waiting. She braced herself, prepared to deal with her reaction, whatever it might be.

CHROMOSOME 17

While chemical interventions and biomedical approaches have been the main research focus in the twentieth century, genetics has become an increasingly greater interest for scientists. Some say that the smaller your topic of study, the more prestige you have. This new subject has garnered massive funding and an equal amount of public attention. Looking not just inside the body but within the tiniest units of humanity could hold the key to treatments and interventions specified to each person. The idea that drugs, food, and every other kind of consumer product could be developed for each individual, accounting for their particular genetic makeup, is alluring. What this approach misses, however, is the fact that genes do not function in isolation of their environment. Genetic mutations that are the cause of illness are generally triggered by something in the environment, either in utero or during a person's lifetime. Without knowing what triggers a genetic change, knowledge of genes may be useless.

Despite this, medical claims based on genetic explanations of disease are considered especially credible and bear more weight than their counterparts (Conrad 1999). Breast cancer exemplifies this. The discovery of the BRCA-1 and BRCA-2 mutations in September 1994 was the apex in celebrating an understanding of breast cancer genetics (Wooster et al. 1994). More than forty-five researchers had been looking for the gene for four years, searching through 600,000 letters of genetic code on chromosome 17. Mary-Claire King, a scientist at the University of California, Berkeley, discovered the association between chromosome 17 and heightened breast cancer risk in 1990, instigating the race between Myriad Genetics Inc., the University of Utah, the National Institute of Environmental Health Sciences, Eli Lilly, and McGill University to find which gene on the chromosome was responsible (Angier 1994). Once Eli Lilly bought the rights to Myriad's genetic tests and therapies, the question seemed close to being solved. Soon enough, it was. Myriad found the gene first, calling it BRCA-1.

The scientific frenzy around BRCA-1 and BRCA-2 was motivated by more than detached inquiry. Patenting such a discovery could lead to enormous profits. The discoverer of the gene would be able to charge any researcher or institution that wanted to use this genetic information in further research. With such a large number of cases of breast cancer every year, this is a potentially mammoth market. Since its patent, implying ownership by the university and Myriad, the gene has been licensed for use by other researchers; meanwhile, fees for its usage build in profits for the "owners." However, the amount of money each institution collected has been kept a secret. The question of ownership of genes is a huge issue itself. Many argue that the most basic components of life should not fall prey to the practices of the free-market system. While the capitalistic spirit has won out in the United States, other governments have ruled against patenting genetic material. European countries have disallowed the practice of economic gain through the ownership of genes, consequently discouraging this type of scientific crunch.

Excitement about the discovery of the BRCA-1 (and soon after another BRCA-2) genetic defect ensued immediately after its discovery. Wen-Hwa Lee, the leader of a scientific team that discovered how the BRCA-1 gene got "lost," hence causing cancer contraction, stated that the genesis or prognosis of "most" breast cancers involved the mutated gene (*Cancer Weekly* 1995). If true, this would mean that a genetic intervention could slow the epidemic. But soon after, scientists began to respond that genes may not be a critical mechanism creating breast cancer tumors.

Since then, the genetics argument has deflated in the scientific world while maintaining public salience. Scientists now agree that genetic causes account only for some 5 to 10 percent of all cases (Davis and Bradlow 1995). Having the genetic mutation also does not mean that a woman will definitely get breast cancer. An estimated 55 to 85 percent of women who have BRCA-1 or BRCA-2 get breast cancer (Milliron and Merajver 2006). Other scientists argue that genetics cannot explain why breast cancer rates have increased in such a short period (Davis and Webster 2002). In addition, twin studies, which are generally scientifically respected as a good test of evidence for genetically related disease causation, show that there is a real lack of evidence to support a genetic argument (Lichtenstein et al. 2000), and groups of women with historically low rates of the disease also develop the same high rates when they move to America (Deapen et al. 2002). Their genetic information must be triggered by an environmental factor. Even when a woman has a defective gene, she can do little now to prevent affliction outside a prophylactic mastectomy, a measure that some high-risk women take.

Even in the 1970s, the early days of growing awareness about breast cancer when the public knew little about it, 70 percent of women knew that family history meant increased risk (National Cancer Institute 1987). In reaction to the massive body of research that had been accumulating since the first genetic study in 1926, David Anderson (1976), the head of biology at the M. D. Anderson Hospital in Texas, wrote, "This type of result is not indicative of a strong hereditary effect" (5). Tracing the rise of twin studies, Anderson continued that the data from twin studies was "suggesting that genetic factors play a relatively small role among all breast cancers" (9). The National Cancer Institute (1987) published an authoritative guide to breast cancer resources that pointed out that "some 'hereditary' breast cancers may actually result from a family's exposure to environmental factors" (5).

A massive amount of research is dedicated to exploring how genetics is linked to breast cancer. It is a part of the biomedical model. Controversies have arisen around the great financial investments being made in an area of research that may benefit only a very small portion of the population: the group that can afford its testing. In addition, questions about what causes genetic mutations have arisen. Women with breast cancer have become involved in research in order to shift the focus, that is, to make research relevant to their concerns.

GIVING THE POWER TO WOMEN WITH BREAST CANCER

As science pursues better treatments and genetic causes, seemingly with no bias and isolated from influences outside the lab, breast cancer advocates host rallies and walks for awareness. The third wave of breast cancer activism made blatantly political moves to change the landscape of the illness. It grew to fund research and shape government plans. Such organizations began to take shape in the early 1990s. They were more political than their predecessors and expressed dissatisfaction with the slight progress made with the disease. Anger was evident. Looking over organizational documents and the little that had been written about breast cancer activism, I found that the largest of these more political groups was the National Breast Cancer Coalition (NBCC). It had played an important role in putting breast cancer on the political agenda. I wondered how it had become political when other organizations were focused on support groups and when there was a serious lack of recognition for women's health. So I traced documents backward to the initiation of the organization.

In 1991, when the NBCC was first founded and the third wave of activism began, other organizations were simply desperate to get women mammograms, access to services, and more humane medical treatment. None had yet attempted to shape research or politics. More than twenty-five years after breast cancer had first been publicized by Happy Rockefeller, Amy Langer, Susan Love, and Susan Hester formed this new kind of breast cancer organization meant to influence politics and gain more funds for research (Stabiner 1997). The NBCC aimed to influence government. These women soon found themselves constantly on Capitol Hill, working many hours for no pay to form the President's Initiative on Breast Cancer.

Following a conference on women and cancer, this group of advocates met to discuss how to begin to deal with breast cancer. Their first concern was the incredibly small amount of funding devoted to the disease. They were also concerned about environmental causes of the disease. Later, this concern got pushed to the margins as more mainstream concerns were addressed. The group, then led by Susan Love, author of the best-selling *Breast Cancer Book*, initiated a campaign that leveraged the moral overtones that mothers make most effectively. They contacted activists from the 1960s, women working in hospitals, and any organization they thought would have some interest and started a Do the Right Thing campaign.

White for the president, green for the Senate, yellow for the House—women all over the country wrote letters to their political leaders, and each group of letters was a different color. The letters were gathered state by state and taken to the White House, where they planned to give the batches to the first President Bush. Marlene McCarthy, a breast cancer survivor with two daughters who ran the first community breast cancer program in Rhode Island, went to drop her letters off. Marlene is a pleasant, feminine woman who nonetheless walks and talks with a purpose. But her assertive presence and the 6,000 letters she carried were not enough to attract the attention of someone from the West Wing or the Capitol. There were no representatives or even aides available to meet with her. "If you leave all that stuff here," the security guard said, it'll be sent down the conveyor belt to the incinerator."

A few hours later, she found herself on CNN deploring her reception with, still, no response from the White House. Marlene recounts, "This was not about me and my breast cancer. This was about the fact that I have two daughters. It's like these little smoldering embers left from the Vietnam era suddenly burst into flames again and the activist was reborn." Returning to Rhode Island, she put together the Rhode Island Breast Cancer Coalition, affiliated with the NBCC.

On October 18, 1993, Fran Visco, the president of the NBCC, presented President Bill Clinton and First Lady Hillary Clinton with 2.6 million signatures supporting the formation of the National Action Plan on Breast Cancer. Bill Clinton's mother had recently had a recurrence of the disease, and Secretary of Health and Human Services Donna Shalala promised that the small budget for breast cancer research would be increased. Even with these promises, it was not guaranteed.

Other activists had convinced two key politicians to be the main support-
ers for breast cancer research. Senators Al D'Amato and Tom Harkin cham-
pioned the cause, Harkin being the first to ask Congress to donate major financial support and D'Amato the second. The key was to find a pot of money
and put it in a safe place where budget cuts could not affect it. The Department of Defense (DOD) was already the peculiar home to a small amount of
money for women's health research. In 1993, Harkin was able to capture a
majority of congressional support for $210 million to be funneled into a new
program for breast cancer research, with the money controlled by the DOD.
The department was the perfect place for any money threatened by budget
cuts since most politicians are loathe to take resources out of defense. It was
odd: women's health was going to get its first real support, with advocate say
on how it got spent, in the most male-dominated governmental agency.

Dealing with health research was difficult for the novice DOD, and the
agency was afraid that other activists might follow suit in hiding research
money in its coffers. It attempted to hand control over to the National Institutes of Health, whose National Cancer Institute made an unsuccessful play
at acquiring power over the funding. But activists intervened. Women like
Fran Visco felt that breast cancer research had not lived up to what was
needed and that the only way to improve the situation was to create an entirely new mechanism of support for research where activists would have a
role in making decisions about the areas studied. Their perspective was not
unfounded since in 1991 there was still no serious breast cancer research plan
(Stabiner 1997). Known as one of the more conservative agencies, the National Cancer Institute also faced the criticism of following a narrow trajectory of breast cancer research. Activists wanted innovative approaches. The
only possibility was a different institute.

As president of the then-burgeoning NBCC, Fran Visco soon became one
of the most powerful leaders in the struggle. Fran was a breast cancer survivor. Her broad smile and dimpled cheeks convey sweetness and docility.
Being the leader of a large organization representing diverse perspectives ne-
cessitated some level of graciousness. But as a former lawyer, the language
she used was specific and direct. Fran knew the vocabulary of law and science. Possessing that power, she appreciated the need that many other breast
cancer advocates had for that knowledge.

Today, Fran's organization encompasses more than 500 groups across the
country. It has three main areas of concentration: research on breast cancer,
access to medical resources for all women, and influence of women with
breast cancer on policy decisions. It has major political influence and has exercised that sway in the legislative arena. Advocates from the organization sit

on the President's Cancer Panel and the National Cancer Policy Board, among other panels, and testify in front of the House, the Senate, the President's Cancer Panel and other governmental agencies. Politicians are not afraid to ally with the NBCC; it represents a national constituency on a bipartisan issue.

As the third wave of organizations like the NBCC developed its constituency and influence in politics, a fourth wave of women was pushing not only for more research but also for science of a particular kind. Activists of the NBCC had been groundbreaking in making advocates review research proposals and open up funding mechanisms for breast cancer—a tall order in itself. They had not made demands about new kinds of research. This new group both benefited from and had to work against what Fran and her colleagues had done. They were less interested in finding a cure. They wanted to find the cause. And they were quite sure that the culprit was in the environment.

CAUSES, NOT CONSEQUENCES

Most say that Rachel Carson was one of the pioneers of environmental activism that linked toxins to illness. Carson, the famed author of *Silent Spring* and the woman credited with initiating the modern environmental movement, died of breast cancer in 1963. She had published *Silent Spring* only one year prior. In it, she claimed that cancers were a direct result of industrial chemicals. She was prophetic. Today we are certain that this is the case, so regulatory caps are put on the release of these substances. This is meant to reduce our exposure to those chemicals to a level that will not be harmful to health. Many claim that regulations still allow too many cancer-causing substances whose effects aren't really known to reach women in particular.

Around the time *Silent Spring* was published, when the United States was newly ensconced in the magic of plastic and other modern man-made innovations, one in twenty women got breast cancer by age eighty (Evans 2006). Back then, black-and-white television commercials portrayed small children joyfully playing in the DDT fog that spewed from the backs of trucks. In these ads, families picnicked serenely as DDT was sprayed under their wooden tables, the haze surrounding them as though it had been accidentally displaced from a horror movie set. These ads were a representation of reality where people were unafraid of exposure to chemicals.

Chemicals are ubiquitous in our environment. Eighty thousand chemicals are currently in use today. Approximately 2 percent of them have been tested for safety (Kroll-Smith et al. 2000). The American public unknowingly absorbs many more chemicals. For example, farmers spray pesticides on crops. As consumers, we know little about which fruits or vegetables are contaminated. Chemicals in the same molecular family make our plastics tough and our nail polish malleable. But we cannot see them. They are often not even listed in the ingredients. Only at times when we have our lawns sprayed for weeds or take a birth control pill in the morning are we aware of the chemical concoctions that permeate our lives and our human tissues. Since the production of industrial chemicals in the 1940s, a long list of compounds has been more subtly injected into our bodies, making some people wonder if the current breast cancer rates are correlated to the spiraling proliferation of chemicals in our everyday lives. Meanwhile, the DDT leftover in American production has been shipped to malaria-ridden countries where it is sprayed profusely.

Scientists conducted a few studies of environmental causes of breast cancer in the late 1970s and early 1980s. Since then, the number of such research projects has grown. However, these projects are smaller in numbers and scientific respect than those looking at genetics, lifestyle, or biomedical mechanisms, such as cell proliferation. Environmental studies are harder to conduct, are harder to draw conclusions from, and therefore win fewer prizes and gain less of the elusive grant money on which scientists depend. The other types of breast cancer risk factors being researched are more accepted in the scientific world. Consequently, these kinds of studies are more common. Doctors usually have little knowledge of environmental health concerns (Brown and Kelley 2000), and the medical advice they do give to women is usually based on more predominant breast cancer research. As a result, the majority of guidance relates to these factors.

Since the turn of the twentieth century, medicine has largely ignored the context from which disease emerges, like the air and water or the politics that shape an individual's experiences (Tesh 1988). There are numerous reasons for the difficulty of environmental research. It is difficult to recount them all. The list of possible exposures is endless—toxins in air, water, food, and makeup. People being studied have no idea *how much* of each toxin they have encountered, much less *when* it happened. So little is known about each chemical that even if researchers had all that information, it would be almost impossible to figure out which one or ones were the reason for an illness. Disease could strike because there are too many in the body or because of two particular toxins mixing together in the blood. In addition, the link between an exposure and breast cancer outcomes has to be high in order to detect an effect. Finding such an association can be difficult when we are chronically exposed to many chemicals at low levels.

When officials at the National Institute of Environmental Health Sciences decided to fund a new study to assess possible environmental causes of breast cancer in 2002, they knew the challenges. The premise of the research was the first problem—to identify what in the environment could be causing breast cancer. Zena Werb, professor of biology at the University of San Francisco, decided to answer this question by picking a number of chemicals that women are exposed to and injecting them into mice in her lab. Werb is a surprisingly well-dressed scientist who could almost never be characterized as having a "bad hair day" like many of her colleagues.

"By seeing how the mice respond," she says of her project, "we can better understand what these exposures mean for women." Her office is located on the thirteenth floor of a nondescript building on the university's campus. A technician walked me from there to the mice lab situated in the basement of a nearby building. These miniature research subjects were stacked on shelves in yellow plastic containers. The technician opened one and removed a mouse for me to observe.

"See this one," he said pointing at a bulbous shape that pushed out of the mouse's side and slid under his finger. "It will die in about six weeks." Gesturing at the others, he added, "They are all at different stages of development." Growth of tumors in the mice would help identify which chemicals are causing cancer in women and how much of each it takes to get there. This type of study takes traditional methods that most scientists trust and uses them to pick out large-scale exposures of chemicals circulating in the environment that could be causing illness and death to thousands of women.

If Werb and her team find a link between a certain chemical and tumor growth, there could be major ramifications for polluters. Research like hers places responsibility on companies that produce chemicals and government agencies that should regulate them. Without studies like it, preventive measures for breast cancer would continue to lean heavily on diet and lifestyle rather than protective measures meant for the larger population—exposures that are small and hard to see but that add up over time. In this way, biomedical research often keeps prevention and causation in the hands of individuals rather than placing responsibility on polluters or regulatory agencies like the Environmental Protection Agency and the FDA, the supposed watchdogs for the American public.

The National Institute of Environmental Health Science is one of few sources of support for work outside the biomedical model. On the other hand, research dollars for genetic and other individual-based research is common. Funding is possibly the most important way the current research agenda is maintained. Because big business provides more research support than pretty much anyone else, many suggest that pharmaceutical and chemical industries can drive the research agenda. Their interests keep breast cancer research focused on profitable and unchallenging aspects of the disease, such as devel-

oping breast cancer treatment drugs or understanding which genetic mutations are linked to cancer whose copyright could lead to billions in profits.
This funding paradigm forms an almost impenetrable barrier to new types of
research. It has led to results about diet and lifestyle but a minimal understanding of causes.

THE MANY EXPOSURES WE FORGET

Chemicals and radiation surround us every day, but we give them little
thought before we are faced with an illness—tingling fingers, a coughing fit,
or cancer. But scientists have been investigating many exposures for some
time. There is a vast and conflicting body of research that connects women's
exposure to specific groupings of chemicals with breast cancer risk (Dorgan
et al. 1999; Guttes et al. 1998; Hoyer et al. 2000). Initial studies showed support for a connection between the chemicals and risk increase. One of the earliest to show a direct correlation between breast cancer and DDE was that of
Mary Wolff and colleagues (1993). This conclusion was based on her landmark study, the first large-scale environmental research project pertaining to
the disease that drew major scientific attention. Since then, an increasing
number of studies have focused on this group of organochlorine pesticides
used particularly since World War II. Some of that research, like later work
by Hunter and colleagues (1997) as part of the Nurses' Health Study, has cast
doubt on Wolff's original conclusions. Wolff and many other scientists still
maintain that there is a link that is important yet difficult to study. Wolff et al.
(2003) argued that "environmental factors are believed to explain much of the
international variation in breast cancer risk" (289).

Ionizing radiation is the only broadly accepted environmental cause of
breast cancer (Boice 2001; Boice et al. 1996). Unfortunate human experiments like women being exposed to the radiation in atomic bombs dropped
on Hiroshima and Nagasaki offered some of the few opportunities to show its
threat. When radioactive material permeated those cities, millions of people
were impacted. While some were so close they were immediately killed, others survived, only to get breast cancer later. Increases in rates in those cities
provided scientific proof that radiation causes cancer.

While debates over which exposures count most—which chemicals, how
much radiation, and the sources of both—evidence about geographic concentrations of illnesses provide the basis that our surroundings influence health.
Women in the industrially polluted northeastern region of United States have
rates elevated above most of the rest of the United States (Kulldorff et al.
1997). Concentrations of breast cancer on Long Island, Cape Cod, the San

Francisco Bay Area, and other specified locations also demonstrate that place influences risk. Marin County, a beautifully landscaped suburb just north of San Francisco, is home to the highest rates of breast cancer in the world (Clarke et al. 2002). Long Island's rates approach those of its West Coast competitor, with rates in some areas exceeding 200 percent above the national average. Another famous vacation destination, Cape Cod, has rates similar to those of Long Island, about 20 percent above their state's averages, which are above the national average (Silent Spring Institute 1998). Researchers are now investigating what causes these breast cancer hot spots, with local environmental exposures being a major component under surveillance.

As early as 1973, studies showed that changing location could impact breast cancer risk (Buell 1973). Asian women provide one of the best examples. Those who reside in East Asian countries have the lowest breast cancer rates in the world. However, data show that the risk for Asian women who move to the West increases 80 percent in the first generation and that the rates for their daughters approach U.S.-born women (Stellman and Wang 1994). While some researchers argue that this is caused by changes in diet, others claim that increased exposures to environmental toxins are to blame. Marian C. Johnson-Thompson and Janet Guthrie (2000) from the National Institute of Environmental Health Sciences suggest that "this shift in breast carcinoma incidence rate as a function of geographic location offers one of the most promising avenues for discovering environmental components of this devastating disease" (1225).

However, like the complications with detecting which chemicals have entered a woman's body, immigration research is difficult to conduct. People in the United States are highly mobile. Children easily move several times before they head off to an entirely different area to attend college. After finishing their studies, they often become urbanites for a period of time before finally settling down in a suburban sector, possibly nowhere near where they were born and first raised. Most studies are not longitudinal and so do not detect this lifetime of movement (Ambrosone 2001; Colditz and Rosner 2000; Greenwald 1999). Those rare research projects that do attempt to tie history of migration to breast cancer have found support for environmental surroundings influencing the risk (Barbone et al. 1996).

WORKING WOMEN

Occupational studies have often found the most blatant support for environmental causation of breast cancer (Labreche and Goldberg 1997). These projects may capture information about chemicals that dissipate quickly and hence are missed by studies that use blood or tissue samples. But there are not very many studies of women in the workplace. Men were considered the most important subjects until recently since scientists believed that women engaged in less dangerous fields. Occupational studies have often taken a backseat to other kinds of studies, like those that examine tissue or blood samples. They have consequently not been counted in the scientific body of evidence supporting an environmental causation hypothesis. While occupational studies were conducted earlier and have been more generally supportive of an environmental causation hypothesis, they have tended to receive less attention in the scientific community.

One of the first studies to show that women were exposed to hazards in the workplace was that of young women who painted luminescent numbers on Timex watch faces (Clark 1997). A nuclear ingredient called radium was mixed with others to make the numbers glow. The workers with their hair tied back and dressed in aprons dipped their brush in the liquid and occasionally in their mouths to make a finer point of their paintbrushes. Soon after, they began dying of head and neck cancer. If those watches are laid on X-ray paper even today, they create a dark mark. Even sixty years later, Geiger counters still detect the radioactivity of the watches.

Further studies have connected occupational risk with breast cancer specifically. One scientist (Hansen 1999) looked at a group of 7,802 relatively young women employed in industries using organic solvents (e.g., textiles, chemicals, paper and printing, metal products, and wood and furniture). He found that increasing duration of employment was associated with greater risk of breast cancer. Among those employed ten years or more in a solvent-intense industry, on average the risk of cancer doubled after ten years of exposure. Another recent study showed a connection between agricultural and manufacturing employment in which women were exposed to chemicals and increased breast cancer risk (Thomas et al. 2001). More occupational research is also currently being conducted by analyzing breast cancer incidence among farmworkers who are regularly exposed to carcinogenic chemicals in the fields (Johnson-Thompson and Guthrie 2000).

Perc is another chemical that women are exposed to in the workplace and at home. This cute nickname stands for a group of liquid solvents whose longer name is percloroethylene. This group constitutes 80 to 85 percent of all chemicals used in dry cleaning. Perc can be inhaled directly, like from dry-cleaned clothes hung in the car or worn the next day, or taken into the body when, after disposal, the chemical finds its way into the ground and then inside fruits and vegetables and ultimately our bodies. Governmental agencies (Occupational Safety and Health Administration 2005) say that short-term exposure causes dizziness, headaches, or unconsciousness and that long-term effects are as serious as cancer. Workers who press dry-cleaned clothes, causing Perc-filled steam to billow into the air, are at particular risk. The Occupational Safety and Health Administration (2005) has attempted, with difficulty, to figure out how to reduce worker exposure to Perc. As a result of suspicions about Perc, the states of California and Oregon have banned the use of the chemical.

ESTROGENS AND BREAST CANCER

Many of the chemicals women are exposed to at work or at home are estrogen mimics that act like hormones in the body. One of the first scientists to discover the impact of hormones on development was Fred vom Saal. His research explored how the feminization of male mice took place in the womb when the mother was exposed to inordinate amounts of natural estrogen. He proved that the most miniscule extra amount of estrogen can influence development in utero (Colborn et al. 2002). Diethyl-stilbestrol (DES) was an early test case. DES was a man-made estrogen prescribed for many women during pregnancy to prevent miscarriage and help a baby to be big and strong. Edward Charles Dodds synthesized DES in 1938, and it was announced as a wonder drug. Not until 1962 did the impact of DES on babies become clear. Having a generally more potent impact on females when used early in pregnancy, it caused a rare form of clear-cell vaginal cancer and psychiatric problems. Judith Helfand's documentary film *A Healthy Baby Girl* grippingly portrays the impacts of DES on the daughters of mothers given the drug. At age twenty-five, Judith is diagnosed with cervical cancer and is forced to have a hysterectomy. Her mother feels guilty. Judith deals with the realization that she will never give birth, and together they meet many other DES daughters, some of whom pass away as the film progresses.

Notwithstanding the brutal impact of DES on two generations, it is far from the most common or essential chemical classified as an endocrine disruptor. Organochlorines are a much more common and larger group of chemicals that contain endocrine-disrupting chemicals such as polychlorinated biphenyls, polyaromatic hydrocarbons, DDT (or, more specifically, DDE, the chemical that is left when DDT breaks down), and nonylphenol. For example, detergent breaks down to become nonylphenol. In lab experiments, nonylphenol leaks from the plastic containers to drastically motivate the production of breast cancer cells. As a scientific/journalist team, Colborn et al. (2002) graphically describe in their book *Our Stolen Future* that these nonylphenol molecules travel up the food chain and around the world. Fish and animal sperm count drops, masculine physical and behavioral characteristics decrease, testicles do not descend, immune systems are weakened, penises may be shortened, sensitivity to male hormones increases, and motor, mental, and behavior problems result. Concentration of these bioaccumulative chemicals increases with each step up the chain. Humans are at the top since we consume all animals that build the food chain below us.

These chemicals turn baby alligators and fish from male to female in the Great Lakes region, slow human neurological development, and are concentrated in the bodies of Alaskan natives who eat large fish on a regular basis. In north-central Florida, Lake Apopka was contaminated by a chemical plant spill of dicofol (a pesticide with 15 percent DDT), an endocrine-disrupting chemical. There, male alligators bore what looked like ovaries and penises one-half to one-third the normal size (Guillette et al. 1994). Female ovaries were severely damaged. Other examples of sexually ambiguous wildlife have been found elsewhere (Colborn et al. 1993). Photographs of such mutated animals appear freakish, as though out of a science-fiction film. Other photos call for a sympathetic response. Birds eggs crack before chicks are ready to be born, and their beaks are misshapen, making it difficult to eat.

Organochlorines are one of the hottest topics of debate in *Our Stolen Future* and increasingly around the world. These ubiquitous chemicals reside in our bodies, the soil, and water. There is good reason for this to be the case; organochlorines are used in the PVC piping that often transports residential water supplies, they are in the pesticides sprayed on our lawns or gardens, and they are easily stored in fat tissue. The polyurethane used to coat a dresser or other wood objects accounts for 12 percent of organochlorine usage. The production of pulp and paper uses another 14 percent, solvents 8 percent, and wastewater treatment 4 percent (Thornton and Weinberg 1993), and this is ultimately put back into the mainstream.

The first landmark moment leading to concern about organochlorines' common usage in plastics and other materials took place in the lab of Ana Soto and Karl Sonnenschein in 1991 (Soto et al. 1994). Soto had not long had the title of doctor when she arrived at Tufts University Medical School in the early 1980s as a researcher. She had come from Argentina to study in the United States and had decided to stay in the country to work with Sonnenschein, a man taking an odd and controversial approach to cancer research. Petite with short brown hair, Soto usually sports a florid scarf or skirt. She is a fiery woman whose scientific zeal only matches her travel schedule. Her office is situated next door to Sonnenschein's in the sterile, white anatomy building at Tufts. Shelves are crammed with the typical array of disorganized books, conference proceedings, and pamphlets that most academics keep. Her walls are dotted with more interesting objects. One black-and-white poster portrays the penises of almost twenty different mammals. From largest to smallest, they stand next to one another, starting with the whale, then the pig penis, which is shockingly long and curled like a corkscrew. The human model falls toward the end of the spectrum. Penis size reflects Soto's interest in reproductive disorders and cancers. Her work investigates why sperm counts are dropping and penis size is decreasing and what these phenomena may have to do with rising breast cancer rates.

Tufts University Medical School is situated in downtown Boston near the bus station, entrances to highways 93 and 90, and the ornate red gate to Chinatown. The school houses some of the most prominent medical researchers in the world. Soto and Sonnenschein are some of them, traveling extensively and funded to the tune of millions of dollars. Their lab is extensive: multiple benches seat graduate students and postdoctoral fellows whose cabinets and drawers are chock full of test tubes and petri dishes filled with experiments. Students come to work with them from around the world, and groups call on them for testimony that many scientists have not had the experience to give. The controversy associated with of much of their work has been part of their fame. They have found a number of compelling and disquieting things that have massive social and scientific ramifications.

Soto and Sonnenschein's most controversial results came out in the mid-1990s (Soto et al. 1994). They were conducting a series of experiments examining breast cancer tumor development in cells. A cadre of research assistants harvested mammary tumor cells that they were purposely exposing to a variety of chemical substances, testing which ones would make the mammary cancer cells grow and which ones would not. One day they found some of the cancer cells growing exponentially for no apparent reason. Since the research team had not introduced new chemicals to these cells in particular, they were mystified. They ran tests for known chemical contaminants to no avail. This went on for months, testing and retesting, with no chemical they could pinpoint as the culprit. One day the scientific team began to use an old set of test tubes, and the mysterious cell growth ceased. When they saw the change, the scientists remembered that they were using a new batch of tubes.

Soto contacted Corning, the company that manufactures the test tubes, as well as fiber optics and dishes, with the information. She requested to know what was in the newly manufactured tubes. Corning sent a representative to meet with her, but he refused to reveal what the new ingredient was, claiming it was a trade secret. After four months of experimentation, the two scientists concluded that the tubes contained a chemical in the plastic, nonylphenol, that had not been in the old ones. This chemical was leaching into the liquid containing the cells and progressing cancerous growth (Soto, personal communication, 2004).

Nonylphenols have long been used in many industries—textile processing, pulp and paper processing, oil and gas recovery, steel manufacturing, and power generation. Consumer products, like cosmetics, cleaners, paints, resins, and protective coatings, all contain the group of chemicals. The accidental experiment proved that the chemicals are estrogenic. This discovery was a historic moment in establishing credibility for the hypothesis that chemicals cause breast cancer.

Nonylphenol is a type of xenoestrogen, or foreign estrogen, that acts like estrogen in the body. There are a vast number of other chemicals that act like estrogens. Organochlorines, often in the form of pesticides or plastics, are also xenoestrogens and are highly toxic. They also accumulate in the human breast (Dewailly et al. 2003). These chemicals gravitate to the many fat cells that inhabit the breast. Some of them make their way into breast milk and then down the throats and into the bellies of newborn infants. We have all absorbed these chemicals through various exposures, and so have organochlorines in our bodies. Although breathalyzers are the butt of barroom jokes, it's not so funny to hear that the breath of many Americans emits one type of organochlorine—freon—the coolant used to make air conditioning work.

Controversy and debate have surrounded research investigating environmental causes of breast cancer. The most suggestive environmental studies have been conducted by epidemiologists studying large populations or occupational scientists who find toxins in the workplace (Bu-Tian et al. 2008; Rudel et al. 2007; Goldberg and Labrèche 1996). Finding a cause-and-effect link in these studies is more challenging because it is often impossible to distinguish those people who have been exposed from those who have not. People simply cannot be isolated from their environment the way cells in a lab can be. In scientific terms, this means that finding a control group is difficult since the American population has ubiquitous exposures to chemical contaminants (Centers for Disease Control and Prevention 2003).

Lack of adequate data also makes research about breast cancer and the environment difficult. It is rare that tissue or blood samples will be collected from a large population and held long enough to see who from that group is afflicted and who is not. Recently, a Danish team used a rare group of twenty-year-old blood serum samples to show the adverse effects of some organochlorines on breast cancer risk (Hoyer et al. 2000). With this extensive database, researchers at the Centers for Disease Control found that an organochloric pesticide, dieldrin, caused women with the highest amounts in their bodies to have double the risk of breast cancer. However, such databases are rare, making it difficult to test specific chemicals. Even when these scientists are able to conduct studies, they often get a lot of flack from the media and other scientists for it.

CONTROVERSIES AND BACKLASH

The magnitude of success can often be measured by the size of the backlash. Scientists examining environmental causes of breast cancer go head-to-head with opponents on a regular basis. One of the most outspoken critics is Dr. Stephen Safe, a professor in the Department of Veterinary Physiology and Pharmacology at Texas A&M University. He has been known to accuse scientists interested in investigating chemical links to cancer as having "chemophobia" and to otherwise call that research "paparazzi science" (Safe 1997). Much of Safe's work is meant to be a direct contradiction to the work of other breast cancer scientists who show support for an environmental hypothesis. In 2002, he and two colleagues from the Chemical Industry Institute of Toxicology (CIIT) in Research Triangle Park, North Carolina, published an article aimed at debunking the idea that estrogenic compounds, like many industrial chemicals found in human blood or tissue, could be tested for their influence on health. In the process of arguing against the negative effects of industrial chemicals, he argued for the usage of tamoxifen, a controversial breast cancer treatment drug.

Like many other critics of environmental health research, Safe has ties to industry that, out of self-interest, must defend claims against their products. But Safe denies that industry influences him in any way (Public Broadcasting System 1998). Safe's association with the CIIT is questionable, although even more difficult can be scientists who disguise their corporate connections. The CIIT was founded by eleven chemical manufacturers and maintains an $18 million annual budget financed by them. The depth of the chemical industry's influence on research conducted at the CIIT has been a source of discussion for more than twenty years. But Safe is far from alone. Many other researchers are also funded by industry. Many of these pose only minimal conflicts of interest. But Safe has been of the most outspoken critics of environmental health research, possibly reflecting the agenda of companies funding the CIIT that have helped move toward disproving that chemicals are dangerous to human health (Fagin and Lavelle 1996).

Even with these critiques of environmentally related studies, the National Institute of Environmental Health Science argues that they are "important because none of the currently known risk factors apply in at least 50% of breast carcinoma cases. Women of color might be at particularly high risk for environmentally associated breast carcinoma because hazardous waste sites and incinerators are more often placed in communities of color" (Johnson-Thompson and Guthrie 2000). The few researchers across the country who support this way of thinking have faced many challenges in getting funding to examine environmental risks.

~*o*

"I knew she wasn't gonna die because I couldn't imagine it. Not my mom," said Brittany, Robin's teenage daughter. "My friend at school's mom had it. She lost her eyebrows and her hair." She paused and looked down at the pink carpet. "A lot of people in Long Island had it," she finished quietly.

Robin's treatment was hard for the family. The kids were confused. Little Eddy did not yet know what was wrong with his mom. Tory and Brittany went about their daily lives, spending the night at friends' houses and going to summer camp. But the noise level at home had escalated. Robin and Eddy could keep the kids under control only by yelling. Eddy looked older. His once bulbous stomach had rounded out with an additional twenty-five pounds. But he had started antidepressants, so his anger was more manageable.

Most days after chemo, Robin lay in bed, sometimes getting up to drag herself to the toilet to vomit. The day I followed her to chemo was the fourth round. The first treatment made her sick for three days. Wrapped around the toilet bowl, she had retched for hours even though she had nothing left to throw up. This time the nurse changed the chemical mix to make it easier on her. Finding the right combination of drugs is a balancing act. The seeming science of it is actually an art that takes years of practice and refinement. Treating the specific case without making the patient sicker might take weeks to achieve. For Robin, the fourth week was easier than the last. She lay in bed, sunlight streaming in, and slept. Exhausted, slightly nauseated, but not vomiting.

II

SECTION II

Chapter Four

The New Breast Cancer Concern

One by one, young women from eastern Long Island were being brought into the morgue. Cause of death: breast cancer. The morgue is the stage where the real toll of breast cancer is played out. Most of us never think about this cold place where mothers, sisters, and loved ones arrive after their long struggle with surgery, chemotherapy, and radiation. These women did not necessarily know one another, so no one could connect the dots the way the mortician could. One might say that the mortician started it all, at least when he mentioned these women to Lorraine Pace. Lorraine was a newly licensed real estate agent taking a flight back home to Long Island. After hearing about the deaths, she made an appointment with her doctor and was told that she had breast cancer (Pace, personal communication, 2006).

"That is when I, Lorraine Pace, a typical suburban woman, became an activist," she said. Checking around the community, she found twenty other women who had been diagnosed as well, with several right around her own house. Lorraine lived in a cul-de-sac where pipes ended, leaving unused water stagnant. She suspected that, over time, chemicals concentrated there. Drinking water on Long Island is drawn from a porous aquifer. Pesticides had been sprayed on lawns and golf courses for years, slowly seeping into the ground and possibly polluting drinking water. "We, on Long Island, depend on our underground aquifers, which is our sole source of water. We need to protect our drinking water, our most valuable resource," she claimed. Lorraine went to her kitchen and filled a glass with water from the tap. She held it up to the light. It was discolored and cloudy. She suspected something in the environment, especially the drinking water.

Lorraine has shiny blond hair, expertly curled to match tailored clothes. She walks slowly and deliberately, as though she is thinking through each next move. Alone or with other people, in conversation or silence, she seems to be planning something. Networking, promoting, and making her agenda known are easy for her. Generally direct and businesslike, she usually wears a sharp-edged suit that complements her robust figure. Her Long Island accent is heightened by a nasal tone and sharp tongue.

After the mortician's story and her own detective work, Lorraine suspected that she might be living in an area with high concentrations of the disease. She called the Suffolk County Health Department repeatedly until she got someone on the line. The health official told her that Port Jefferson, where she lived on the northern side of the peninsula, actually had lower rates than West Islip, just to the south. But when pressed for details, the official admitted that this calculation was dated. Shoe boxes of postcards from New York Hospitals reporting breast cancer cases had been sitting in the Department of Health for five years. Lorraine took the situation into her own hands and started what would later be called the breast cancer mapping project.

A cadre of volunteers went door-to-door handing out surveys. They got a 60 percent return rate—high for any survey, much less one done by volunteers. Each positive response they received meant a new pink dot was put on a large white map kept at the office. As Lorraine said, "Every one of these dots represents a woman who asks the question—why? She is one of the millions that want to know why."

"This was done from my dining room table for eighteen months," Lorraine explained. It was an exhausting and ambitious adventure. Lorraine and other women collected information to fill what was a blank slate about how many women had breast cancer. They hoped it would indicate some pattern of who was afflicted and why. Knowing little about how to technically codify this data, Lorraine's group hired a research team from the State University of New York, Stony Brook, headed by Roger Grimson, a biostatistician, to map these cases into a new computer program called Geographic Information Systems (GIS). GIS technicians code data into geographically described units that can then be visually overlaid with other specific locations. Roads, parks, and state lines are some of the most basic. Lorraine's group wanted to know about pesticide spraying by contaminants from Brookhaven National Laboratories, a local military facility, like from the 1930s potato farming that was followed by long-term spraying of DDT, especially in the 1950s.

Lorraine's work captured media attention. She appeared on the front page of *Newsday* with the title "Asking for Answers" riding high over her head. As she picked her way through technical language and scientific methods, Lorraine began to help other groups do the same. Mapping projects emerged all over Long Island and in other states and countries like California, England, and Japan. Activists in Marin County, California, also called to ask for her help in starting their own mapping project. Soon, Marin Breast Cancer Watch in the San Francisco Bay Area was formed on the same premise as Lorraine's group.

Lorraine seems almost like a war hero considering the number of awards and honors she has received since she met the mortician. The list on her résumé is more than a page long: National Organization for Women Community Champion, Healthcare Person of the Year—Suffolk Life, Humanitarian of the Year—Beth Sholom, and Women's History Award. She has met with no less than President Bill Clinton and Hillary Rodham Clinton, senators, state representatives, celebrities, and community leaders and has made appearances in press sources as diverse as *Scientific American*, *U.S. News and World Report*, *Prime Time*, and *Eye to Eye*. She has volunteered as a lay reviewer for the Department of Defense, the National Cancer Institute, and the American Cancer Society and as an activist for the March of Dimes and the local PTA. But Lorraine was only one of several breast cancer leaders on Long Island. As she began her mapping project, other Long Island activists were contacting political representatives to push for government funding for research into environmental causation. They were finding out what they perceived to be heightened rates and wanted to know why.

Long Island was the first place that new science investigating environmental causes of breast cancer was begun—and defeated. While the National Breast Cancer Coalition was developing its constituency and influence in politics, other groups of women on Long Island, Cape Cod, and the Bay Area in San Francisco were all following a different trail. They were the first to begin changing the debate about breast cancer. Although they were largely unaware of all the research that had already gone into detection, cure, and treatment, they quickly found that there were few answers about causes. They wanted to change that. Although unique and groundbreaking in starting a new dialogue about the illness, they faced major scientific and political challenges.

Activists on Long Island began to change science out of necessity. Little research had been done linking environment and breast cancer, and almost none of it addressed the exposures with which they were concerned. Their activism was not directed at any corporations and initially did not even acknowledge that there was a political economy to breast cancer. However, as they shifted the science of breast cancer, the political economy began to follow suit. Responsibility for illness is shifting from an individual locus to a corporate one, where large-scale institutions must take responsibility for the molecules they release into the streams, veins, and air particles around the world. Long Island was the first testing ground for shifting the political economy of the disease.

My first visit to Long Island was in 2000. The graduate school at Brown University had given me just enough funding to get me there and back a couple of times and to take a trip to San Francisco as well. I figured that I had a pretty good deal compared to some of my graduate student friends who were forced to spend the summer straining their necks over test tubes in a sterilized lab. Both Long Island and the Bay Area were supposed to be beautiful in the summer.

On my first trip to Long Island, I took the ferry from coastal Connecticut to the North Shore. I parked my car in the underbelly of the boat and climbed steep stairs away from the gas fumes up to the passenger level. It was still early in the morning, so I bought a cup of instant hot chocolate and took a seat in a shiny, red booth to watch the water below. I must have dozed off because I awoke violently to the brash ferry horn. Long Island arose atop gray-blue water, its landscape fading from green to a pale white sky. Sparks of silver flecked the water as sailboats and dinghies reflected the bright sunlight.

The scene was peaceful. Only a small breeze disturbed it. No clouds of smog hung over the land. I began wondering what had ever made women think that something in the translucent air, crystal-clear water, or apparently rich soil could be making them sick. If nothing else, they were impatient with the years of cancer research that had led to little understanding about causes of the illness, about why it had become so common. They were concerned that a "blame-the-victim" mentality had surrounded how breast cancer is dealt with—that women themselves had to prevent the disease with little thought as to what the factors outside of lifestyle, diet, and exercise might be.

These breast cancer activists argue that environmental factors should be a more noticeable item on the public agenda. At the same time, they claim that preconceptions about the disease are preventing its demise. They have transformed personal troubles into social problems by engaging in a new variation of the classical feminist approach: "the personal is political." Today's breast cancer activists are entirely different from women with the disease even thirty years ago who had little choice but to accept a doctor's opinion. They have questioned medicine and taken their critique a step further in challenging science. They were some of the first to shape women's health research by increasing research funding in massive proportions.

These activists responded to finding out about heightened rates around their neighborhood. At first, they were alarmed. Cancer clusters often initially cause fear, then questions (Brown and Mikkelsen 1990). If a cause can be determined, the ultimate emotion is anger, usually directed at the factory, company, or polluting sources that have long provided jobs while dumping on the community. On Long Island, the cause was not clear. Most of the women with breast cancer they met did not have the traditional risk factors. They had eaten healthy, had children early, and never smoked. The one thing they seemed to have in common was where they lived. They wanted to see research into the potential toxins around them.

Ubiquitous and poorly regulated chemicals were suspicious targets. First, there were emissions from local factories and power plants or pesticides sprayed on lawns and crops. Then there were other endocrine-disrupting exposures that superseded local boundaries: polycyclic aromatic hydrocarbons (PAHs) in air or parabens and phthalates in products like makeup, cleaners, and plastics. Studies show that exposures to these endocrine-disrupting chemicals have special links to cancers of the reproductive system, like breast cancer (Markey et al. 2002). Science has proven that radiation from medical procedures or electromagnetic fields is also cancer causing (Caplan et al. 2000). These exposures are everywhere. Chemicals can be inhaled, absorbed through the skin, or eaten. They're frightening. Other breast cancer activists had ignored them.

Robin pulled on her black ski jacket and pushed the front door open. The ocean breeze had shifted to a sharp, whipping wind for the winter months, and wisps of her blond hair bit her cheeks. I trailed behind her with my camera. She turned out of her driveway and walked slowly down the street. As we left the water behind, she began to point to houses.

"My girlfriend lives there," she said, indicating one across a small inlet. "She's a little younger than me, and I know she's scared." Gesturing toward a brown house even closer to us, she explained that the woman there had been diagnosed with breast cancer a few years prior but that she was not very neighborly, and so Robin did not know the details.

We kept walking. Robin's street emptied out onto a slightly larger road that wound through the subdivision as smaller streets cut away to the left and the right. They all looked similar to me with names like Avon and Devon places and Secatauge and Bay streets, numbers one through eight. Some of them ran directly back to the ocean's edge with lucky home owners who had a 180-degree view of gray-blue water. As we migrated from one street to the next, Robin narrated. Here, one woman had died of cancer. Turning left, another had been diagnosed twice. It seemed impossible. But, in fact, according to some mapping projects on Long Island, these kinds of neighborhoods are not rare. Statistically, they do not amount to much. For those who lived in this seeming oceanside paradise, it was frightening.

CHANGING THE SCIENCE OF BREAST CANCER

In 1991, Barbara Balaban did not have breast cancer, but a lot of her neighbors did. At that point, one in nine women were getting breast cancer nationally, yet around Barbara it seemed like many more. On a regular basis, she received phone calls from friends about yet another woman succumbing to the disease. Barbara knew the area and had lived there a long time watching the Great South Bay's peaceful gray waters while havoc was wreaked in the lives of women on her own block and the adjacent streets. She had owned her home on the bay for twenty-five years and had become a community leader. Lucky for Barbara, the lines on her face and her graying hair had not been prematurely earned by regimens of chemotherapy and surgery. Rather, they denoted the hours and days she had devoted to women with breast cancer, a group whose size she feared was rapidly swelling.

As it turned out, Barbara's suspicions were right. On Long Island, about twenty-five women within each four-square-block radius had breast cancer. Unlike the state of New York's rate of 102.1 cases per thousand, Long Island's rate was 118 (Committee on Science 2002). Only pockets of the island had "expected" rates. Even those were almost always above the national average. The rest of Long Island was covered with what the government called "areas of incidence not likely due to chance" (New York State Department of Health 1999). Barbara ran several support groups and a breast cancer hotline on Adelphi University's rolling, green campus in western Long Island. Other than these services and another advocacy group appropriately termed "One in 9," there was little responsiveness to the mushrooming disease. Few recognized that the ordered suburbs of Long Island were being permeated by a hotbed of breast cancer cell proliferation. Like Lorraine Pace, Barbara was one of the first to draw attention to what she saw: too many women with the disease and no explanation why.

In 1992, a governmental study of breast cancer and the environment on Long Island came out with scientists concluding that no more studies were necessary. This transformed Barbara from a local hotline and support group coordinator to an activist.

"I said there were only three things wrong with that study—the way it was conceived, the way it was executed, and the way it was reported," Barbara protested. "I looked at the women who were coming to the support group, and they didn't fit the high-risk category. So I thought there's something missing, and what could it be? The only thing I could think of was environmental. Everything else was diet, mainly Jewish, old when having had children, or family history. Most people didn't fit that. So the thing we had to look at was where people live and their environment."

From her work on the hotline, she knew who was getting breast cancer. She had worked in the community while surveying the increasing numbers of nearby women with the disease. The claims of the study did not match up with the real picture. Barbara had not been afflicted but did not feel immune to it. On the contrary, she was acutely aware of being surrounded by it. Just like the clam boats that used to dot the bay and had disappeared since there was no harvest, women were dropping out of the community, sick. Increasing pollution decimated the clams and women alike.

Balaban became the leader of a group of activists who wanted to see the environment investigated. She had recently been involved in a National Breast Cancer Coalition meeting where scientists and activists concluded that $300 million would be necessary to develop a real research plan. Now she needed to figure out how much money would be required to study environmental causes of the disease on Long Island, and for that she would need help figuring out what to study. Barbara called Susan Love, who had helped found the National Breast Cancer Coalition, and Devra Davis, the scientist who helped publicize the endocrine disruptor hypothesis.

Davis and Love were the ideal combination of experts—a well-known, cutting-edge researcher and a famous breast doctor—to connect the disease to local concerns. Once the scientists agreed to cochair the meeting, Balaban called researchers all over the country. Twenty-six attended, and together they came up with an idea of how to approach the topic. They needed a variety of studies to examine all the ways in which women were being exposed. Money was the problem. Barbara used her former political connections. As part of her work with the National Breast Cancer Coalition, she visited with longtime New York Republican Senator Al D'Amato. She had heard that he wanted to have the recent study, which had concluded that environmental factors were not important, reviewed by the public. She promised him that if he could get the Centers for Disease Control (CDC) to come to Long Island, she would have at least one hundred residents there to argue for funding a new study about environmental causes of breast cancer on Long Island. He agreed.

The CDC came. The promised residents arrived. Testimonies by women with breast cancer were heard, and, like any political event, politicians gave assurances. Barbara and her friends were not satisfied without concrete progress. They took advantage of the credibility the CDC's visit had given them and pushed D'Amato to write a congressional bill to fund a new study of environmental risk factors that could be increasing breast cancer on Long Island. Although D'Amato was a Republican and the environment a Democratic issue, he jumped at the opportunity to support these women. A longtime political strategist, he realized that their concerns were beginning to span the island. Most were not in politics, but they had money and connections. It was an election year, and he needed their backing.

Public Law 103-43 was passed in June 1993. With support of the National Cancer Institute and the National Institute of Environmental Health Sciences, scientists were mandated to "conduct a case-control study to assess biological markers of environmental and other potential risk factors contributing to the incidence of breast cancer" in Nassau, Suffolk, and Schoharie counties of New York. Project organizers hired a range of scientists from Iowa, North Carolina, Maryland, New York, and California. Congress granted \$32 million for a group of thirteen different projects including two case-control studies to analyze blood samples and exposure to PAHs. Researchers would also look at the impacts of electromagnetic exposures and home pesticide use (Gammon et al. 2002a). The Long Island Breast Cancer Study Project was the first federally funded project passed by Congress stipulating what would be studied and exactly what scientific methods scientists would use. It was controversial and by far the largest research project about environmental links to breast cancer.

Researchers first established registries that kept track of who got cancer and in which county in the area. Then they began to collect new data. Many of these studies used new approaches to understanding risk. One of the most significant projects utilized GIS. In this instance, they overlaid breast cancer cases with hazardous waste sites, industrial facilities, or the toxic release inventory, the governmental measure of where and how much hazards are emitted. The GIS researchers then compared those maps to the layout of drinking water systems to analyze how toxics might have seeped into drinking water and if that might have caused the disease. The bill also supported research on the impacts of electromagnetic exposures, chemical contaminants in tissue samples, and home pesticide use (Gammon et al. 2002b). It was a diverse set of studies that covered a vast scientific terrain.

Women on Long Island were ecstatic, but the challenge was only beginning. For the next ten years, they would struggle with their involvement in the research. They had voiced concerns about drinking water from the study's inception. Lorraine felt strongly that the design of the Long Island piping system meant that women living in cul-de-sacs were drinking dirty water. But researchers thought that other factors, like chemical residues in women's bodies, were more important. A battle ensued over what would be studied and how.

Town hall meetings were held so that Balaban and other people from all over Long Island could offer insight on possible environmental contaminants. Hundreds of local residents gathered in churches and community centers so that Gammon and other scientists could tell them about the Study Project and ask their advice on environmental exposures. Variables for the GIS study were created on the basis of these town hall meetings. The meetings were a way to gather community input and for researchers to feel like they were accountable to the women who had gotten them funding. Meetings with the public had been planned into the initial research plan, but there was no direct translation of local concerns into research questions. An umbrella organization, the Long Island Breast Cancer Network, was the main group working with researchers, uniting the diverse set of local groups—the West Islip Breast Cancer Coalition, the Huntington Breast Cancer Action Coalition, the Southampton Long Island Breast Cancer Coalition, Sister Support, and One in Nine. Off and on throughout the study period, they met with researchers. But in the end, many of the women felt like their voices had not been heard.

With or without debates between scientists and advocates, studies like the Long Island Breast Cancer Study Project that investigate environmental causes of breast cancer are complicated. Calculating the impact of exposures to an endless number of factors is scientifically complex. In one of the Long Island projects, Merilee Gammon and her team tried to isolate whether PAHs were linked to higher rates. PAHs are in car exhaust, pollution from power plants, and the burned edges of a grilled hamburger (Khalili et al. 1995). As in many other studies, the first challenge was simply determining exposure. With a glass of wine per day, that question is simpler. Women can tell researchers how many drinks they generally consume. With PAHs, it is a quagmire of remembering when you ate a hamburger, measuring the air pollution you are generally exposed to, and a number of other factors. Maybe it was the ketchup and not the hamburger that mattered. Or perhaps the vitamin C in the ketchup offsets the damage from the hamburger. To simplify the process, scientists often look at what is in the body. This omits the complexity of many exposures to just what remains in tissue, blood, or urine. In this case, they measured the amount of PAHs in the blood. They found that higher amounts of PAHs were related to higher risk of breast cancer (Gammon et al. 2002b).

Many outcomes of the Study Project appeared to question whether there were links between environmental exposures and breast cancer. But similar to conducting the study itself, understanding the results of studies like the Study Project takes patience and close attention to detail. The most obvious results are not necessarily the most important ones. The devil is in the details. One study concluded that organochlorines, like pesticides, were not linked with breast cancer. However, the story is more complicated than this. Researchers measured the amount of chemicals in the blood around the time a woman is diagnosed with breast cancer. This exam could take place many years after an initial exposure. For example, a woman could have been one of the little girls running behind a truck spraying DDT in her neighborhood who later developed breast cancer. By the time she gets the disease, the amount of chemicals left in her blood might be quite low. But inhaling the spray at a much younger age could have been what flipped the switch to begin development of breast cancer in her body. The disease incubates for many years.

The research team conducted other studies with mixed findings. All of them faced a complicated landscape of exposures, making it difficult to find an answer. Later, the research design would come into question, and blame would be shunted back and forth between the researchers and local women about who had chosen what to study. Lorraine, who had started the first mapping project on Long Island, would be angry about the wrong chemicals being studied, and Dr. Gammon would respond that old pesticides like DDT that was sprayed in the 1950s were ones scientists knew best how to handle. Debates over the science marked time as more women got breast cancer.

TIT FOR TAT

Following in the footsteps of Lorraine Pace, Karen Miller was one of the first to start mapping breast cancer on Long Island. Mapping appealed to Karen not from a scientific perspective but from the artistic eye of an interior designer. A high school graduate who met and fell in love with her husband-to-be at age thirteen, Karen spent twenty-three years in the interior of homes dressing them up. Over the years, her business grew, and her biggest clients became celebrities in the recording industry and Hollywood. She gave birth to three children—a philosophy professor daughter and two sons, one a technical analyst and the younger a Wall Street broker.

A year and a half after getting fed up with the consumerism of her trade and selling her business, Karen had a suspicious mammogram. It was the day before Thanksgiving 1987. She spent the day preparing the next day's family celebration, keeping the news to herself but the thought never slipping out from the back of her mind. Soon, she had to tell her family and have her breast removed. Her surgery took place at Memorial Sloan-Kettering Cancer Center. There, she met other successful businesswomen facing the same malignancy. They formed the "tit for tatters." As Karen phrases it, "having lost a tit, we figured we could tit for tat." The women bonded immediately, meeting every week in either Manhattan or Long Island. Doctors became aware of the group of strong, articulate, successful women and began to refer like women.

The group joined forces with the powerful and influential Barbara Balaban. One in Nine was one of the backbone breast cancer organizations on Long Island, and Barbara ran it smoothly from her base at the Adelphi hotline in Nassau County. But as the group grew and began to contact their local representatives, they knew that a grassroots movement was necessary. Breast cancer was an issue not only in Nassau County but also in West Islip, Huntington, and East Hampton.

Karen called Lorraine Pace. She wanted help in starting to map the cases in Huntington. Lorraine worked with index cards, going door-to-door to survey the 9,000 people in her area. But there were 63,000 households in Karen's town, and index cards would never suffice. Then help seemed to shower on Karen out of nowhere. Her name had been in the *New York Times* and local newspapers, and companies, researchers, and local residents started calling offering resources. Her mapping project grew, as did her name in the community, and soon enough Karen became the first advocate to review grant proposals for the Department of Defense, which had begun funding breast cancer research on a grand scale when the National Breast Cancer Coalition pushed Congress to allot monies to its protected coffers.

Karen did not have any preparation other than reading the huge stack of materials given to her dealing with Dr. Gammon's complex initiative. When first called and invited to be a peer reviewer, she balked.

"I said, 'I don't even understand it, and I think you chose the wrong person. I don't have the medical knowledge, and I'm not . . . ,' I told them everything I was not," recalled Karen. The scientist at the other end of the line said, "Please think about it. If you decide to do it, we'll call you tomorrow, and then we'll give you the stuff." She relented and spent months reading preparatory materials. But she was nervous about being the first breast cancer advocate to advise the Study Project.

It was during these first meetings with scientists that Karen began to advertise the persistence of Long Island breast cancer advocates. The Long Island Breast Cancer Network had just come into being, and she told her review committee about it. Soon the network invited the National Cancer Institute to meet in the polished, lush boardroom of the Omni building in Nassau County. The owner of the building donated the room and catered the network's events. Karen knew the importance of presentation and took advantage of the opportunity to impress the National Cancer Institute, letting the governmental officials know they were dealing with women of influence.

Karen was in some ways unlucky to be first. Later, women would often undergo intensive training about the most technical aspects of the science and biology of breast cancer before being placed on review boards. ProjectLEAD became an important program to offer this service. Since the mid-1990s, when Dr. Kay Dickersin, one of the board members of the National Breast Cancer Coalition, began the program, advocates meet four times a year for four intensive days at a time. During those four days, scientists lecture and quiz women with breast cancer, helping them to understand the scientists' perspective. By the end of the retreat, women who may not have had a science class in twenty years understand the basic biology, toxicology, and epidemiology involved in complex scientific questions (Braun 2003).

Up until the initiation of the Department of Defense project where women with breast cancer became voting members of review panels, scientists were in control of research projects. Advocates joining review panels changed this situation, at least sometimes. Review panels are formal judging mechanisms whereby a group of experts selected by the government decides whether a research proposal should be funded. On these new panels, women's perspectives were first met with skepticism by most of the scientists. Advocate approaches were very different and often meant a serious critique of the science involved. For example, advocates criticized the usage of the p value, the percentage of chance that a hypothesis is false. In the scientific world, the smaller the p value, the more impressive the study. A p value of .05 is often used, but it is not as remarkable as .01, which means that a scientific hypothesis is very likely to be true. Since scientists generally claim that nothing is ever "provable," this is as close as they allow themselves to get to taking one side or another on a scientific finding.

Using the p value means that a very narrow range of studies is judged as finding any outcome. But some scientists claim that a study result greater than .05 is still meaningful. Activists and some scientists publicly argue that the stringent p values being used in breast cancer science undermine support for an environmental causation hypothesis and that epidemiological methods were inadequate to measure the variables they thought important. Scientific constraints such as these restrain the process of reaching a scientific conclusion and therefore often also hold policymakers back from taking a stand.

For Karen, getting involved in reviewing proposals meant that her insight on breast cancer could be felt not only through her work on the Long Island project but also in research happening all over the country. But in both cases, her voice was hard to hear. Surrounded by scientists and few to no other advocates, working on a review board or in a study is tough. Expressing a dissenting voice or a novel idea when the credentialed experts are on another page means that voices like Karen's are not always heard, even when they are present. This was the problem with the Long Island Breast Cancer Study Project.

LOOKING FOR ANSWERS

When Long Island activists pushed Senator D'Amato to put research on breast cancer and the environment onto the agenda, he not only instigated the Long Island Breast Cancer Study Project but also initiated the Program on Breast Cancer and Environmental Risk Factors (BCERF) at Cornell University. D'Amato approached the president of Cornell, Hunter Rollings, to ask for his help in answering the concerns of breast cancer advocates. Since Cornell had expertise in toxicology and there was concern about the role of pesticides and other chemicals, Cornell was an ideal place to address whether chemicals were causing the disease. The president immediately formed a committee to see what Cornell could do. In 1995, BCERF was formed.

Cornell's Institute for Comparative and Environmental Toxicology (ICET) translates research about breast cancer and the environment into accessible information for the public and policy consumption. BCERF is housed under ICET. Although the acronym BCERF, pronounced "Be Surf," suggests New Age–type meditation on ocean waves, the organization's work is strongly rooted in the facts and figures of the most up-to-date science. Through research and meta-analysis of published research, this group assesses potential environmental causes, such as pesticides and other chemicals, in addition to more traditionally researched topics, such as diet (Warren and Devine 2004). Public education by BCERF includes a quarterly newsletter and an extensive website that provides information on scientific studies, the evaluation of potential breast cancer causation by various chemicals, and breast cancer mortality maps. A cross-disciplinary group of staff works under the rubric of BCERF, ranging from medical professionals to risk management experts.

BCERF sits at the crossroads of breast cancer organizations, scientists, and companies. Community groups, advocates, policymakers, scientists, and public health professionals meet several times a year to inform its work. Its purpose is to identify areas of potential collaboration, inform policy, and generate new ideas. It is an important and challenging position to hold in the landscape of breast cancer research. Such a vast amount and diversity of scientific work is conducted that it is difficult to keep up with it, much less look at it in a comprehensive way and translate it to the public.

Suzanne Snedeker is the associate director for translational research at BCERF. She possesses, perhaps, the most up-to-date knowledge on research about breast cancer and the environment of any researcher in the world. After working with the BCERF program since its inception in the mid-1990s, Snedeker recently wrote, "It is unfortunate that the media has given the impression that few environmental factors have been associated with human cancer. The World Health Organization's International Agency for Research on Cancer (IARC) has identified 80 natural and synthetic chemicals, occupational situations, pharmaceuticals and viruses that cause cancer in humans." She continued, "We cannot paint the picture of breast cancer in a single stroke. Rather, each study contributes a small piece to the mosaic of breast cancer risk. Each piece starts as a question, a hypothesis, based on the best information available at that time" (Massachusetts Breast Cancer Coalition 2003).

Although Dr. Snedeker has broad knowledge of chemicals in our environment that may cause cancer, her knowledge—and ours—is limited by the reporting of polluting corporations by government agencies. As Suzanne reports, there are no databases that list all the chemicals being used in industrial processes, and it has been incredibly challenging for her research institute to develop its own list. One research assistant spent an entire school semester on this task, only to come up short—and frustrated. The most reliable source of information is in the National Toxics Program, which has concluded there are forty-two chemicals circulating in the environment that cause breast cancer (BCERF 2004). Nonprofit groups, like the Environmental Working Group in Washington, D.C., that specialize in finding hidden environmental data are another source of assistance. But no matter how much detective work Snedeker and other organizations carry out, there are still gaps in understanding what chemicals are out there and their effects on the human body.

FINISHING THE LONG ISLAND BREAST CANCER STUDY PROJECT—SLAMMING THE ACTIVISTS

It took ten years from the start of the study for the results of the Long Island Breast Cancer Study Project to be published in a scientific journal. As soon as they were released, the press started to pick up on the results. The *New York Times*, the *Los Angeles Times*, *Newsday*, and a slew of local newspapers began regurgitating the same outcome, one following on the heels of the next, simplifying one another's work by repeating the same conclusion over and over: there was no evidence of environment being linked to breast cancer. The presses slammed Congress, the scientists involved, and activist groups for the way the research was done. *Newsday* claimed that "political pressures, inflated expectations and the competing demands of activists and scientists have conspired to undermine the [study]" (Fagin 2002). In a similar vein, the same author reported, "Even though some researchers and news reports warned of the immense complexity of the science involved, they were outshouted by groups willing to encourage such outsized expectations."

It was the first major study of environmental causes of breast cancer where activists were involved. These women with breast cancer had gotten the congressional funding for the Study Project and tried to shape the way it was done. This amount of nonscientist input was unprecedented and, to some using their twenty-twenty hindsight, a mistake.

Gina Kolata (2002), the science writer for the *New York Times* who most frequently covers breast cancer, was one of the loudest voices in discrediting the study. In her article titled "The Epidemic That Wasn't," she quoted an epidemiologist saying that "it is an example of politicians jumping on the band-wagon and responding to the fears of their local population without really thinking through what is going on in science." This was not the first time that Kolata had downplayed the links between environment and breast cancer or diminished the role of industry responsibility. She had been at the *New York Times* since 1987 and in 1988 reported on big tobacco. Then she (1988) had claimed that "industry documents never show that the tobacco companies had definitive evidence damning cigarettes." It was as obvious then as it is now that the companies did have definitive evidence. Because of that knowledge, they lost the largest class-action lawsuit in history (Givel and Glantz 2004).

In 1995, Kolata was awarded the Sound Science in Journalism Award by the corporate front group Advancement of Sound Science Coalition (Source-Watch 2006). Two years later, she reviewed a landmark study by David Hunter that concluded that chemicals have no effect on breast cancer risk. Kolata (1997) reported that "one more environmental scare bit the dust last week as scientists from the Harvard School of Public Health reported that their large and meticulous study found no evidence that exposure to the chemicals DDT and PCBs [polychlorinated biphenyls] are linked to breast cancer." Her article ignored the six other studies released around the same time that did find evidence to support environmental links to breast cancer (Aronson et al. 2000). Perhaps she did not have the background about them, or possibly she ignored a lot of the evidence.

The scientific and media response to the August 2002 publication of the Long Island Breast Cancer Study Project (Gammon et al. 2002a, 2002b) was exceedingly sharp and appeared to be more an attack than an objective discussion. Critics claimed that the negative results from the Study Project demonstrated both that environmental causation is not a useful research direction and that public participation is dangerous for science (Fagin 2002).

Despite the one-sided view offered by the press, some scientists celebrated the scientific merit of the study. Julia Brody, the executive director of the Silent Spring Institute in Massachusetts, pointed to one of the studies showing that women with the top 25 percent of PAHs in their tissue had a 50 percent increase of breast cancer risk. This finding validated twelve previous studies. Well-known scientists like Dr. Brody; James Huff, director of the National Toxicology Program; and Lorenzo Tomatis, former head of the International Agency for Research on Cancer, opposed the media backlash. But no newspaper published their op-eds or even letters to the editor. Why that happened is an important but possibly an unanswerable question.

Getting the Study Project going had taken a lot of work, and results had been a long time in coming. The idea of the Study Project began to form in 1991, and the public did not see the study's results until 2002. During those eleven years, women on Long Island had joined together to lobby politicians and draw public attention to their hypothesis. Long Island women faced institutional and scientific challenges when it came to the Study Project. Activists wanted to shape the research agenda of the projects. But by the time they got their hand in, much of the research methodology had already been designed and the variables to be studied selected. As a result, the public was consulted only after the majority of the projects were planned. In the end, they had little influence on most of the studies, and advocates felt that many of the things they wanted addressed were excluded. For example, they requested that chemicals currently being used, such as pesticides, plastics, and cosmetics, be studied. Scientists instead chose to study PCBs like DDT and chlordane, whose usage had been curtailed years ago. Scientists selected these chemicals because they are easier to detect in the blood and body fat than many others. But their lack of contemporary usage made it close to impossible to know either the time of exposure to the chemicals or the amount of chemicals women had absorbed. None of this was accounted for in the media coverage. Consequently, the public walked away thinking that, as usual, there were no environmental links to breast cancer.

As the Study Project progressed, other research investigating environmental causes emerged around the country, spurred on by other activists who wanted more research on environmental causes of breast cancer. All of them had faced the same challenges in initiating studies and stood to encounter similarly harsh criticism on completion. The largest such endeavors were four Breast Cancer and Environment Research Centers funded by the National Institute of Environmental Health Science and the National Cancer Institute at $150 million. These centers spanned the United States, making use of the most renowned research institutions and universities. Other smaller projects had also popped up in California and Massachusetts.

Two fallen bicycles lay next to the driveway. A basketball had rolled into the grass near them. I tapped on the front door and went in. There was silence. A moment of play seemed to be interrupted, stopped in time, suspended. The living room floor was covered in toys and the kitchen counter stacked with containers and packages. Robin called from upstairs that she would come down. Otherwise, the house was devoid of its normal hubbub with the kids at summer camp.

Chemotherapy had been hard on the family. Things had gotten messy and relating to one another even more difficult. I had come that afternoon to talk to Eddy to hear the man's perspective. I could hear the shrill ring of Robin's cell phone upstairs and her muffled voice answering. She emerged at the top of the staircase a few seconds later. Eddy was on his way back from the office. "I am sorry I didn't do anything to myself," she said. She was wearing glasses, which I had never seen her in before. They had heavy black plastic frames that shadowed her blue eyes. Her hair, with its long brown roots, was pulled into a loose ponytail. She wore no makeup. Her tone was lower than I was used to. She seemed tired. She had just finished chemo.

We could hear Eddy approaching, talking rapidly on his cell phone as he opened the front door. He came in and sat down while Robin worked on preparing dinner. I asked him if we could talk, and he agreed. He moved from a stool at the counter to a wooden dining room chair near the end of the kitchen just within Robin's earshot. He began talking, at first haltingly, about how it had been to watch her go through treatment. He was deeply tan at this point in the summer and had gained weight that bulged from under a baby-blue T-shirt. His baseball cap covered damp black hair that only peeked from under the edge.

"My wife kept saying I had anger management problems and that I was acting different, but I couldn't tell. We went to the doctor, and he gave me something that, after a few weeks, I felt really different."

"Yeah, you stopped yelling so much," Robin added from the counter on the other side of the room. "He wouldn't even talk about it with me."

"What? We talked about it all the time," Eddy responded. Robin came and sat at the table with us.

"You said you wanted to do it nine to five."

"Yeah, it was like a job to me. Nine to five, then we could enjoy ourselves the rest of the time and not think about cancer."

"This was the worst, most horrible thing to me," Robin looked at me. "My partner, my best friend wouldn't talk to me about what was going on with me."

"I would, just nine to five," Eddy said, lifting the cap and wiping his forehead with the back of his forearm. Eyebrows raised, he looked first at Robin, then at me. "This is the first I have heard of all this."

They both looked over my shoulder to something behind me. Little Eddy was standing there looking at us. He had come in without us noticing and had been listening, who knows for how long.

"Come over here and give me a kiss," Eddy said to his son. Little Eddy walked over, and the three broke into everyday conversation. What had happened at camp? What are we having for dinner? I sat back and watched. A veneer of normalcy descended on the scene covering what had been exposed, if for only an instant, in front of stranger's eyes. Conflict was hidden to the rest world but not from the family, I was sure.

Chapter Five

Fresh Evidence

The locals are dry mouthed and chapped even in the summer as they wait for another windy, deserted winter. Many describe the land they live on as jutting out bravely into the ocean like a flexed arm that ends in a clenched fist. The peninsula of Cape Cod almost floats on water, only a shallow bed of sand separating it from the depths of the ocean floor. Local drinking water is drawn from a porous aquifer like that of many ocean-bound lands, Long Island included, transmitting a diverse array of particles from Hyannis to Provincetown. Cranberry bogs have flourished here for years, emerging like a red mold from the earth at harvest time. Raised like rice in watery marshes, cranberries thrive in colder, aqueous environments. This all-American traditional Thanksgiving garnish attracts insects when humid cape summers arrive. Farmers spray pesticides profusely to ward them away. Toxic chemicals land on the plants and in the water, sinking into the receptive ground that waits to transport it to drinking water.

The spraying and porous aquifer may be the partners in crime responsible for excessive rates of breast cancer on the cape. Other potential culprits are a military base that has emitted radiation and other airborne chemicals or the PVC piping that leaches carcinogenic remnants into drinking water. Few cape vacationers are aware of the cancer proliferation in their sun-drenched destination, and with cape businesses depending on tourists for their livelihoods, no one is talking.

Even under this curtain of silence, women in Massachusetts have generated new insight into what could be causing the heightened rates of breast cancer on the cape. Their work has a ripple effect across the scientific community. In Long Island, researchers and activists studied some of the same exposures as previous researchers and were attacked for their work. Massachusetts activism started with the same premise as that of Long Island—that environmental exposures needed to be better understood—and then moved in a new scientific direction, studying factors that had never before been looked at. Worried that the results might generate panic or overwhelm its underfunded agencies, the researchers' work has caused government suspicion. In some ways government concerns are justified. The results have long-term ramifications for how agencies regulate and what we do about breast cancer.

Massachusetts is home to some of the most groundbreaking work that has shifted the scientific economy of breast cancer. Researchers changed the fundamental tools of science to replace those often inadequate to understand environmental links to the disease. These tools are adept at capturing evidence never seen before. Information has been literally pulled out of thin air—the dust, particles, and other exposures that hang there, historically unstudied but always absorbed—demonstrating new evidence about what women face every day. New evidence is shifting the ground that researchers stand on, mounting in ways that were previously impossible. Such scientific change in Massachusetts has led to innovation in other places. And maybe more than that, it has given concerned women credibility in pointing to weak toxic regulations and even weaker political representatives. As a result, new legislation and laws have been passed. Steps have been taken to slow the constant deluge of chemicals in the environment. But before all this was achieved, there were just a few women who even thought of *causes*.

Cheryl Osimo is a cape resident who once had no knowledge of breast cancer rates in her area. That was until she became a victim. In her early fifties, Cheryl's olive skin has retained the vibrancy of youth. Her straight hair is short and practical, and her makeup is minimal like the classic Massachusetts woman. Cheryl is more open than the typical New Englander, using a quick tongue to exercise her sharp wit. The rapidity of her speech only begins to attest to an endless stream of energy carrying her from one person to the next in any social gathering. The root of this energy seems to be an enduring love for others and a great sense of justice. She exudes support and warmth.

Usually bright and lucid, her dark eyes only dim in telling her story. "I was really very healthy," Cheryl began. "I was doing really well. I exercised. I wasn't overweight. I ate all the right foods." Knowing what was to come next, she paused a minute. "I thought I did all the right things, and then I found a lump. I went for a mammogram, then I went for an ultrasound. They told me I had a suspicious lump. Eight months prior I had been give a clean bill of health. I said to the doctor, 'I know there's a lump, and that's why I'm here, and do you think I should have it out?' The doctor said 'Is it bothering you?' I said, 'No.' He said, 'Well, then why take it out?' So I didn't. Eight months later, I have this 2.5-centimeter infiltrating ductile carcinoma with lymphatic vascular invasion; terrible prognosis.

"I went into surgery to have a lumpectomy, and they did the operation. The doctors went in thinking they were just taking out a negative tumor. I remember they sent a piece of the tumor in to do a cold-section biopsy, and the pathologist called. I heard the phone ring, and I heard him say, 'Oh, uh-huh.' I didn't hear him say, 'Oh good,' and I knew. I just knew. I sensed something was wrong. And there was a young intern with dark eyes, with dark-rimmed glasses, he had to have been in his twenties, and I remember him looking down at me with those deep dark piercing eyes, and he looked at me, I looked up at him, and he had a tear in his eye. I remember seeing one tear coming down his eye on his face, and I said, 'I have cancer, don't I?'

"I'll never, I feel like crying every time I talk about it. I don't tell many people. I don't usually share that with anybody because it's too hard for me to say.

"As I laid there listening to the doctor and technicians talking, it became clear to me there was a question about whether or not they would be able to take the tumor out within the margins. I said, 'If you are going to get close to the margins, cut my breasts off.' I became an immediate behavior problem on the table. He said, 'Cheryl stop, you don't need your breasts cut off. Your breasts are big enough. I can get clean margins around the tumor. I'll just cut the tumor off.' I said 'No, I want it cut off. I want it cut off.'"

Soon after Cheryl went into a deep depression, a dark hole, as she describes it. A friend called and invited her to a meeting of the Massachusetts Breast Cancer Coalition (MBCC). With cajoling, she agreed to go. It was rare for Cheryl to venture outside her world, her house, her day care, her husband, and her kids. The women met in a small room at Burger King. They spoke openly about their breast cancer or the experiences of loved ones. Unlike most groups that were largely about support, this one was made up of activist women who focused on prevention. They not only wanted to support each other in getting through treatment but also were looking for a way that other women could avoid getting breast cancer. Cheryl pulled herself together and was invited to join the board of MBCC and a few years later she founded Silent Spring Institute, a research group working closely with the Massachusetts activists. She soon became coordinator of the Cape Cod office. Before she found the lump, Cheryl did not go out much. Today, she speaks at Rotary Clubs, Lions Clubs, Kiwanis Clubs, women's clubs, colleges, and business and professional women's organizations to talk about prevention of breast cancer.

"I know that I am doing my best be a part of the movement to change the world, to make it a better place not just for my children or my grandchildren but for future generations," she said. "I can't sit here. I couldn't have gone on with my life as a teacher or a day care provider and just keep going on in my life as I did with my head stuck in the sand ignoring everything that happened."

TURNING THE TIDE

Soon after activism emerged on Long Island, women in Massachusetts joined in. Although Massachusetts women did not know about what had been happening a few states over, they were all driven by the same goal—not just to find a way to cure breast cancer but also to prevent it. Along with women on Long Island and in California, the MBCC was one of the first to remake the breast cancer activist agenda.

I began to learn about the history of the MBCC from Deb Forter. Deb is a tall woman with a distinct sense of style, a broad forehead, and gentle eyes. Her easy laugh and fluid leadership style suggest many years spent in California. She had been referred to the MBCC by the National Breast Cancer Coalition when she moved back to Massachusetts from the West Coast. Just prior to her move east, a friend of hers died of breast cancer. She began volunteering in her memory. At that point, the Massachusetts group was inexperienced but not untested. It had recently gained state funds to initiate a research institute looking at environmental causes of breast cancer on Cape Cod. But the research they had initiated was controversial and was threatened at every turn by its funder. Deb was critical to holding things together.

After almost six years of volunteering, Deb became the codirector of the MBCC, based in Boston. By then she had adjusted to the East Coast, the cold weather, and the time-consuming work of activism. During that time, the organization moved from cramped quarters in a western suburb of Boston to a spacious office in a brick building in the southern region of the city. Over the years, Deb grew into the humble force behind the organization now focusing almost solely on possible environmental causes of the illness. It lobbies politicians, holds fund-raising events, and offers educational workshops about how to decrease personal exposures to toxins in the home and work.

"I think that activists have been the ones pushing the rock up the hill," she said to me when we first met. "They became very vocal and held rallies and got women empowered to do something about the high rates. And as a result of that, they did get the legislature to declare that breast cancer was an epidemic in Massachusetts, which was very unusual."

As the MBCC developed into a powerful entity that legislators paid attention to, it joined with other health groups. The Women' Community Cancer Project was the most political. Lise Beane had been a cofounder of the organization. Lise lives on one of the most beautiful historic streets in Boston. Almost fifteen years ago, on this tree-lined avenue where some of the oldest money and bluest New England blood resides, Lise became a breast cancer activist.

"Ten years ago we were this desperate circle of women sitting around in a dimly lit room. Many of the people had cancer, or relatives had cancer, or friends had it, and lovers," recalled Lise. "We began to tell our perspectives. I remember my sister saying before she died that the strength of the future was communicating to people what you do well and what you don't do well. I thought that was like a little message from her. So one of the things we did was stand up and tell what we do well and what we didn't do well so that we could ascertain our strengths and weaknesses. There was an epidemiologist, a biologist, a social worker, and then they came to me and I was a copywriter and visual person with a background in design and visual communications."

Unlike the modest Deb, Lise is a fast-talking Bostonian. She figured out how to market a cause. Lise designed the public outcry that helped the MBCC pass the bill for environmental breast cancer research. She designed color-coordinated outfits to unite the women in the pivotal rally in 1993 that led to enough public support that the state congress passed the bill.

The rally took place on a cloudy Boston day. Shoppers walked through the area in typical northeastern dress—blue jeans, black shirts, warm hats, and clunky shoes. The marchers were notably different. By the hundreds, they walked through downtown Boston in hot pink T-shirts with black lettering. They carried posters and chanted.

"Forty or fifty signs I hand lettered, fueled by the sickness of my sister dying in my face. It was my only way of getting out the pain. I would say, 'You haven't seen anything yet.'" The plaques read, "What's killing us? We demand to know the whole truth" and "Breast cancer and the environment— Make the connection."

As they reached their destination, the famous and touristy Faneuil Hall in downtown Boston, the women filled an open space in a small amphitheater. There, Lise had drawn the outline of Massachusetts. March leaders asked women in the audience with breast cancer to step into the outline. Slowly they filled the oblong space. In that moment, a fraction of the endless numbers of women with breast cancer in Massachusetts flowed across the edges of the state, united by geography and their similar experiences. Hundreds of women, many with breast cancer, looked each other women in the eye, recognizing the pain they had endured, seeing the strength that they still had.

Lise explains that her work "is not just about breast cancer. Breast cancer is just a wedge issue. If we can change the way the world sees this disease and how it treats women with this disease, then we change the universe of women's health."

Katie Richards* was one of the women who stepped into the chalked outline on the black concrete. She was forty-two when she was diagnosed with breast cancer. Like most women when they are first diagnosed, she was no activist. She was a doctor, trained at Tufts University and practicing psychiatry in Boston. Yet the mental challenges she underwent postdiagnosis—denial, grief, and anger—were ones she did not anticipate. Soon after she began to accept her diagnosis, Katie sat in the bleachers of a breast cancer rally in Boston. It was a typically cloudy summer day. What made it different were the hundreds of women dressed in bright pink shirts carrying placards and banners on the street below.

The rally organizers asked all women with breast cancer to come out of their seats and step into the map. "So many people came out of the stands, I couldn't believe it." Katie said. "Young women, old women, black women, white women. I was flabbergasted. It was at that point that I said to myself, 'When I went to medical school breast cancer was rare.' I'm forty-two. I don't have a family history. I suddenly have breast cancer. I'm looking around at hundreds of women who have breast cancer, and this isn't rare." That was 1991, the same year that she joined the Board of the MBCC.

The next year, in 1992, the Department of Defense (DOD) initiated the Breast Cancer Research Program, run under the Congressionally Directed Medical Research Programs (CDMRP). True to its title, the program was created so that Congress could mandate certain types of health research. During the first years of its existence, the Breast Cancer Research Program (BCRP) was meant to support research on screening and diagnosis for military women. But when Long Island activists pushed legislators to fund research into environmental causes of breast cancer, all that changed. In the following ten years, Congress appropriated a total of $1.4 billion for research on breast cancer and other illnesses (CDMRP 2003).

The research supported by the CDMRP was peer reviewed. This type of research, which requires proposals to be evaluated by a panel of experts for their merit, was not unusual. What was striking was the inclusion of women with breast cancer on review boards. Activists had demanded that they be able to influence what research was done, and Congress had mandated that advocates sit on panels that reviewed DOD-funded scientific proposals. In the

---

*Names have been changed to protect the anonymity of the participants.

words of the program itself, the BCRP was meant to be "a partnership of consumer advocates, clinicians and scientists collaborating with the DOD to identify gaps in research design, new mechanisms for supporting research, and guide the funding process." This was the first time in history that Congress had mandated nonscientists have the power to influence the relevancy of research.

Suzanne Snedeker, from Cornell University's Program on Breast Cancer and Environmental Risk Factors (BCERF), explained, "You have to credit the breast cancer organizations for really opening up and changing things to have survivors involved. Now, for any foundation or major granting organization, it is considered critical to have disease survivors on the review boards. That was totally unheard of fifteen years ago. It was the DOD that really cracked that. There isn't an organization I can think of that doesn't have lay reviewers." She continued, "The National Institute of Environmental Health Sciences has cancer survivors involved in an ongoing basis in all aspects of the research. They are involved at an extremely high level. That is a huge impact cancer survivors have had on the process. A lot of cancer advocates have learned how hard it is to do science. The scientists have benefited from the survivors, and the advocates have learned about the scientific process as well."

Katie was like Karen Miller, one of the first to work on the review process. In 1996, Katie, along with another MBCC member, served on the DOD peer review panels. After being selected that year, the two women were sent ten to twenty proposals each and asked to submit detailed written comments on them. This was no small task. Even though Katie had medical training, she found it challenging. Once she reviewed the proposals herself, analyzing the topic, methods, and overall relevancy of the research, Katie convened with the whole advisory board. Around fifteen people, almost all of them scientists, sat in a room together, debating studies and deciding their fate. The group met for prolonged periods of time, generally a long weekend where they would enter a room first thing in the morning and not leave until the sun had long set and their eyes were watering with fatigue. After the weekend ended, the group would turn their evaluations of the studies over to the DOD, which would make the final decision about which to fund.

Running peer-reviewed research involves a lot of people and is complicated. Involvement of activists like Katie makes it even more so. There are two kinds of involvement by nonscientists: peer review and programmatic review. Peer review is the first-run judgment on the technical proficiency of a scientific proposal. Then the cream of the crop goes on to the programmatic review, dealt with by the integration panels. These panels are composed of scientists, clinicians, and two advocates. Scientists who are on those boards are the tops in their field and know the full gamut of research in their area. Advocates on integration panels are selected to have a national perspective that reaches outside their own experience and communities. These panels attempt to answer complex questions about how funding can be balanced in different areas by cutting up pieces of the research pie, optimizing research dollars, and not letting all the funding go to one field.

Governmental institutions that do peer review are accustomed to dealing solely with the scientists. Scientists are selected on the basis of their professional credentials—their degrees, current place of employment, publications, awards, and so on. Picking advocates is more difficult, largely because the selection process is new and may be more subjective. How do you decide which woman with breast cancer can best represent the experience of having breast cancer? The National Cancer Institute (NCI) faces this question every time it picks participants for a new panel.

The NCI is one of the largest government health bodies to use public participation on a broad scale. It even organizes it for the DOD. Two companies run advocate involvement for NCI. United Information Systems oversees most of the peer review process at NCI—the proposals, panels, consumer reviewers, and logistics. The company interviews women with breast cancer over the phone to make sure that they have a broad perspective and are representing experiences other than their own. Scientific Application International Corporation does the other half of the peer review work. Once a year, it negotiates the nomination process and sends out application packets to advocacy support groups and organizations all over the country. Organizations' leadership selects members from its constituency to be recommended.

I began learning the details of women's involvement in peer review boards the summer after my second year of graduate school. I was commuting between Providence and Newton, Massachusetts, four days a week to work at Silent Spring Institute. Newton is a beautiful suburb of Boston, unfortunately unreachable by commuter rail from Providence. There, in a short brick building on the first floor, worked a research team made up of hydrologists, public health researchers, Geographic Information System (GIS) experts, and statisticians. I did not have the mathematical or scientific backgrounds they had. I had been brought there to study how breast cancer advocates took part in their research—how effective the collaboration was and what kinds of changes they made in science. That I could do.

What made learning about the DOD, NCI, and CDMRP review process interesting was being able to compare it to that at Silent Spring, an organization not run by the government. Like the CDMRP, Silent Spring had been instigated by activist concerns about breast cancer. In both cases, women with breast cancer, many of whom were not scientists, were given a seat at the table where new science is developed. The CDMRP put a few advocates on a review panel and let them battle it out with a large number of scientists who knew a lot more than they did and who did not necessarily care about their input. Together, the review panels would look at proposals that had been submitted by researchers all over the country. They were responding to a request issued by the government that mandated what would be studied and often the methods that should be used. As a result, advocates could only say yea or nay on particular proposals. They could never truly shape what would be studied or how. Some argue that this format disempowers advocates while making it look like the government cares about their opinions.

Silent Spring was different. The advocates who had pushed the state of Massachusetts to give the scientists funds to found Silent Spring were directly involved in generating new research questions and methods. They asked questions: Why were there high rates on Cape Cod? Could it be the military reserve? Are there toxins in my home? And the scientists tried to figure out how to answer them. It was an entirely different model, and it seemed to be creating much more revolutionary science.

WACKY GIRL SCIENTISTS

When alone, they joke that others see them as "wacky girl scientists." If seen in the grocery store or headed to work in the morning, they do not look wacky, dressed in modest skirts or slacks, no dyed hair or much makeup. But in the scientific world, those from traditional institutions see them as truly experimental. Julia Brody, the director of Silent Spring Institute, is one of their leaders. Her organization is the only one anywhere devoted solely to studying the relationship between breast cancer and the environment. She is serious and relentless in her quest both for good science and for accountability to the public. Her ethics are embedded in deep knowledge of the impact that industry-funded science has on knowledge of breast cancer and her belief that research should be unbiased.

Brody grew up in beautiful Washington State in a small town down the highway from the Hanford Nuclear Site. Every day as she entered school, she walked by a banner of a mushroom cloud, a testament to the power and danger of the facility nearby. Some afternoons when alone in the house, Julia would answer the phone to hear the Hanford nuclear emergency phone droning the monthly "red alert" practice, "Please stand by for roll call!" This monthly test and the nuclear threat were a part of normal life, much as the growing number of cancer deaths was becoming routine to people across the country. When her father died of cancer at age forty-eight, the hazard that had seemed in some ways so far away became closer to home than Julia had ever imagined it would.

In her second job after college as an environmental reporter and then during her graduate work in environmental psychology, it became increasingly clear to Julia that often the causes of environmental problems and cancer deaths were obvious. But getting people to take care of the obvious problem was a political challenge. In other cases, where science remained uncertain, it was pushed aside and trivialized rather than vigorously pursued. Often the powerful interests that caused the problem would attempt to make the threat seem like a far-off hazard. She began to learn more about how people psychologically distanced themselves from the increasing number of potentially risky technologies that they encountered every day. She saw how individualizing environmental protection by putting on safety gear made this distancing process easier, hence slowing political action that at-risk groups might take. She noticed that both this public perception of risk and the way that science portrayed it was pivotal to either generating or slowing political change. She began to believe that risk perceptions were pivotal in influencing what questions were studied and the scope of ignorance. So when Brody became the director of a research project where researchers and activists banded together to investigate possible environmental causes of breast cancer, it was no surprise.

Earlier breast cancer research in Massachusetts had paved the way for Brody's institute. In 1991, Boston University scientists Ann Aschengrau and Dave Ozonoff began to examine the incidence of nine cancers in Massachusetts (Aschengrau and Ozonoff 1992). Dry-cleaning facilities in wealthy areas like Newton had turned out to be surrounded by cancer. They had also found that people living near the gun and mortar positions of a local military reserve on Cape Cod had increased rates of breast cancer. The Canal Electrical Plant and Pilgrim Nuclear Station, hubs of energy for the cape, were also contaminated sites, but the cape was generally still a mystery.

That year, the MBCC was founded. It was the first activist group to pursue environmental causation of breast cancer in the area, despite the high rates. In part, MBCC activists were responding to the rates on Cape Cod. On that sunny peninsula, breast cancer incidence was—and still is—20 percent above the state average (Silent Spring Institute 1998). A map of the state with county-level breast cancer rates outlined is almost all one bland color other than a few dots around Marblehead and a bright band of color reflecting heightened incidence on the cape. Nine of fifteen towns in the state with heightened rates are situated next to one another on the cape with rates increasing the more distant they are from the mainland.

The MBCC had become a thorn in the side of several state representatives. Representative John Klimm and Senator Therese Murray from the cape area were told about the rates on the peninsula that had been significantly higher than the rest of the United States since 1982. The MBCC jump-started Silent Spring Institute in 1994 by pushing a bill through the Massachusetts legislature. The bill provided $1 million a year for research about environmental causes of breast cancer on the cape. Unlike the Long Island Project, Silent Spring's plan was built on activist and scientist collaboration. They meant to not only develop new science but also educate the public about possible environmental causes of breast cancer. Members of the MBCC would travel throughout the cape and the wider state, holding workshops in homes, community centers, and schools. Silent Spring began to host events throughout the year, such as the annual "Swim or Walk Against the Tide." Members of the MBCC advised the research process as members of the institute's Board of Directors and Public Advisory Committee. A team of renowned scientists composed the Science Advisory Committee as the alternate component to the Public Advisory Committee. It includes the institute's staff scientists and coinvestigators from Boston University, Harvard University, Tufts University, and other research groups. The researchers both advise the Silent Spring scientists and educate MBCC activists about research proceedings.

The first phase of the Silent Spring study was completed three years after the institute was founded. Through this first project, the institute began establishing its role as an innovative and controversial group of scientists. Most basically, it created a detailed surveillance of breast cancer incidence (Silent Spring Institute 1998, 2000). The researchers developed a massive body of data in its GIS that mapped the homes of 280 women on the cape, half of whom had breast cancer and the other half who didn't (Brody et al. 2002). The scientists then overlaid sites of environmental contamination, such as where pesticides were sprayed or chemicals had been released, with these data points. This was the first comprehensive picture of how many women on the cape had breast cancer and where they lived. This picture was meant to test the idea that women who had breast cancer were being exposed to toxins, possibly causing cancer.

Brody's team also tested traditional risk factors like family history. Scientists had also claimed that increased usage of mammograms might explain why rates seemed to be higher. Neither of these factors explained why average rates across the cape were above even the already high U.S. rates. "Our research has found that the elevated breast cancer incidence is indeed a longstanding problem for Cape Cod, and one that is not easily explained by established risk factors, such as reproductive and family history," stated the final report published by Silent Spring in 1998 (Silent Spring Institute1998, 2). The task of the next four years was to figure out the missing pieces of the puzzle. After giving their preliminary report, their primary funder, the Massachusetts

Department of Public Health, removed support. It was post-9/11, and states were facing major fiscal crises. Either that, or the department just didn't want to get caught in controversy. Meanwhile, Silent Spring began to slowly regenerate federal grants to finish the analysis.

PUTTING THE PIECES TOGETHER

Initiating the second half of the cape study meant facing scientific challenges in order to answer hard questions. The first phase of the report had established that rates were high and had eliminated suspicions about traditional risk factors. It also began to show some links to specific contaminated sites. The research team began innovating new scientific methods that could pick up data most researchers ignored. Ruthann Rudel, one of the senior researchers at Silent Spring, pioneered much of these inventive approaches. Rudel has boisterously curly hair and a dry sense of humor. She is staid, precise, and mathematical like most scientists, but her background is a bit more diverse, including training in neuroscience, chemistry, and environmental management. In her case, multidisciplinary training has led to novel thinking and new scientific tools.

Rudel, Brody, and their team decided to collect multiple types of data. Since drinking water was a way that toxins could be transported and consumed, the team developed an extensive history of pesticide use and drinking water quality on Cape Cod. The second phase also involved interviewing 2,100 cape women. Brody and Rudel's staff asked these women about environmental toxins they may have been exposed to either at home or in the community. For example, some have used pesticides on their lawn, while others have seen them sprayed to rid the area of gypsy moth, mosquitoes, or other pests in the home. Many of the chemicals tested are endocrine-disrupting chemicals and mammary carcinogens (Rudel et al. 2001). Reports from individual women were then combined with estimates of environmental exposure using the data from GIS mapping (Brody et al. 2002; Silent Spring Institute 1998). Since much of the existing science about causes of breast cancer relates to family history of breast cancer, reproductive history, and use of pharmaceutical hormones, the researchers gathered this personal information and included it in the final analysis.

I went on a research trip with Ruthann and her coresearcher, a former college baseball player. They were returning to a home of one of the 180 women on the cape who had breast cancer and had agreed to let them collect samples inside her home. The one-story white house we visited did not stand out from the others on the windy gravel road that led down a hill, approaching the ocean. The backside of the cottage was mostly glass, offering a panorama of sea framed by bright blue sky and sea grass. Lydia* and her husband Sheldon had lived in the house for more than thirty years. They had raised two daughters and still had the cribs and dollhouses in a back room to prove it.

Rudel was going back to the house to pick up the data collected by an air monitor in the basement, to collect dust samples again, and to report back to the couple what the research team had already found. At first, she and her assistant collected another layer of data in an attempt to understand the source of some of the more surprising chemicals. In order to collect more dust, Rudel's assistant inserted a small white tube into a typical vacuum. When the vacuum sucked dust out of book pages and off the backs of bookshelves, the dust collected in the tube. It was then carefully removed and laboratory tested for chemicals. He also removed the filter in an air sampling machine. This would give information about what airborne exposures the couple was facing.

Since only certain chemicals could be found in the samples, Ruthann took more time to ask painstaking questions about what chemicals got used in the house. Spray deodorant, lawn pesticides, cleaners, new furniture with factory-made fixatives in the cloth—she asked about a broad array of suspects. Rudel examined each room of the house with the family, looking at each piece of furniture, asking about when was it bought, and finding tags that indicated its ingredients.

Pulling all of the data together, the team found thirty chemicals that women were encountering and that scientists had never realized (Rudel et al. 2003). Some were discontinued long ago but still remained in household air. Unlike the Long Island project that studied chemicals out of usage, the Silent Spring Institute examined both past and current exposures. Chemicals like DDT and flame retardants have long since ceased to be used in the United States. But they are still in the blood of cape residents. The researchers also tested for phthalates, pesticides, parabens, alkylphenols, polybrominated biphenyl ethers, polyaromatic hydrocarbons, polychlorinated biphenyls, and others. They found eighty-nine endocrine-disrupting chemicals either in the bodies of cape residents or in their homes. Fifty-two compounds were found in the air of cape homes. Sixty-six were in dust and twenty in urine. Most of these endocrine disruptors had never been studied before. The most common were products from plastics, personal care products, and cleaning products. In many cases, the levels in homes exceeded existing federal safety guidelines.

Some of the chemicals Brody and Rudel (2003) found had no guidelines for how much can be in the body or home without being harmful. Since most of these chemicals are used outdoors, government regulators never thought that they would creep indoors where they would be encountered day in and day out. Manufacturers did not realize or at least did not care that their products would get in the body and stay there. But as Jack Spengler, a member of Silent Spring's advisory board and a professor at Harvard University School of Public Health, said in response to the findings, "We were surprised to find remnants of chemicals like pesticides and flame retardants that have been banned for decades in dust and air of Cape Cod homes. Some of these chemicals do not break down easily indoors, so *we should be concerned about what gets into our homes in the first place*" (Silent Spring Institute 2006, 14, emphasis added).

Before leaving the couple, Ruthann sat down with Lydia at the kitchen table to explain a sheaf of papers seemingly full of bar graphs and indistinguishable chemical names. Sheldon peered over their shoulders. The papers contained the results for what had been found in their home. A new chemical was represented in a graph on each page. Small empty circles ran up the left side of a bar graph representing the amounts of chemicals the research team had found in the home on their last few visits. If available, the safe level developed by the Environmental Protection Agency was represented by a short line drawn at an interval along the bar. Page after page, the group looked at each chemical. Lydia asked Ruthann about what each level meant and where the chemical could have come from. Ruthann answered. Reporting the chemicals in their home to the couple was an ethical challenge. There is little solid understanding of the link between specific exposure levels and risk of illnesses that the chemicals are known to cause.

Hours and hours of questioning and collecting, observing, and investigating paid off. In the end, Silent Spring's methods made headlines. The *Salem News* (2005) declared, "Dust study shows toxins are right under our noses," and the *Boston Herald* said, "Tests find toxins in Cape homes' air" (Caywood 2004). Their findings spread through the scientific community showing that studying the experience of women in their day-to-day lives was quite different than most breast cancer research. By innovating new methods, the researchers were able to conclude that hormonally active agents are common even indoors. Establishing the existence of these chemicals is the first step to creating broader scientific study and pointing to the need to regulate them.

Brody's team focused only on Cape Cod. But how different is the cape from other places? Silent Spring Institute compared its results with studies done in other areas of the United States and found that some chemical levels were higher on the cape and some higher in other locations. In other words, each place we live has distinct risks. But chemicals are everywhere. Mary Wolff, one of the first and most famous scientists to investigate an environmental link to breast cancer, said in response to Silent Spring's findings that "the products we use in our homes for cleaning and personal care as well as the materials used to build and furnish our homes all contribute to the chemical mix in which we all live" (Silent Spring Institute 2006, 16). We are all swimming in that morass. It is just a matter of how much we face and when we get exposed.

ROBIN'S MOVE

Robin was getting better, regaining strength, and beginning to get back to her normal life. She seemed calmer, slower than when I had first met her the summer of her mastectomy. Maybe she was just more resolute. The kids had returned to their previously rambunctious but relatively behaved state, bickering with one another but stopping before Robin had to scream at them. Renovation of the house was back in action, and the compact structure now looked like its face had been ripped off with the pale wood inner framing only partially covered by new siding. When I arrived for my last visit with Robin, the front door was temporarily missing, and a chilly breeze blew into the house. Robin was in the kitchen using a new matte silver toaster. She wanted to tell me about their future plans.

"We are moving," she said. This was the first I had heard of it. I was surprised. I thought they were investing in the house in order to stay, not to go. "I just don't want it to be because of the environment. Maybe it's safer in Connecticut." She was carrying small piles from place to place, and heaps of papers and toys were scattered around the living room, where afternoon light washed over the gray carpet. "And Eddy wants to start some business there. It just makes sense." I was, in fact, not sure that it did make sense for them to leave if their motivation was escaping exposures that could have caused her cancer. Rates of breast cancer in Connecticut are not that much lower than on Long Island, and as I had learned from research on Long Island and Cape Cod, toxic exposures are everywhere.

I could not tell her this. Their plans were already being made, and my opinions and advice were not important. I wondered if she would feel safer there, if moving away would allow Robin to leave her experience with breast cancer behind and start anew. I hoped so. For myself, I had realized some time ago that there was no real safe place to escape to. There was no bubble I could crawl into. I knew that I had to make the world safer. If I didn't do it in my own way, no one would.

Chapter Six

Under the Skin

Andrea Martin grew up in Tennessee and stayed in the South to attend Tulane University in New Orleans. Petite and quick to smile, she fit the southern belle look, if not the attitude, a soft persona that hid an inner resiliency—an iron fist in a velvet glove, as they say in those parts. She earned a master's degree in French at Tufts University in Boston, then moved to San Francisco to teach. She quickly dropped that to go to law school and get married. After getting her degree and practicing for several years, she returned to her southern roots, buying and managing a Tennessee-style barbecue restaurant, Hog Heaven. Her marriage had gotten into trouble, and she needed to get out of the restaurant business. She also had to earn enough to support her young daughter, Mather.

Single again, Andrea was not alone long. Her second husband, Richard, came along, and she sold the Hog to raise her daughter. They had been married a year when, in 1988, Andrea was diagnosed with stage 3 breast cancer. It had spread to her lymph nodes, and she was given very little time to live. "I was basically told to go home and put my affairs in order because it was already stage 3 and had gone to my nodes," Andrea described it. With one breast removed, she underwent a year of intensive treatment: sessions of chemotherapy, sitting in a chair with a needle in her arm administering the drugs, followed by nausea and vomiting. Her daughter and husband had to cope with a different Andrea. But she survived, at least temporarily.

Four years later, Andrea discovered a lump in her remaining breast and received her second grim diagnosis. It was scary, the unnatural ball-like feeling of a growth in otherwise soft flesh. Last time, she had been terrified. This time, she was pissed. It was only two months into Diane Feinstein's campaign for Democratic governor of California. Andrea had been working on the finances for her. When that race ended in defeat, Feinstein appointed Andrea deputy director of the northern Californian part of her run for Senate — a bad time to get sick again. It meant taking time off from the campaign to have her second breast removed.

"At that point my fear turned to anger," Andrea said in describing the experience. "Very little was still being said about breast cancer. The Komen Foundation had been around eleven years. They were doing great work, but they were very polite and didn't make much noise. It wasn't really an advocacy movement because it isn't an advocacy organization. I thought that we needed a strong national organization that was pushing the edge and constantly questioning the status quo rather than going along with it." After the surgery, she made an assessment. The National Breast Cancer Coalition was the only really political breast cancer organization. And there seemed to be a lot of sick women. It was time to found her own organization.

"Breast cancer turns all of us into activists one way or the other," Andrea said to me, leaning forward in a large leather chair that dwarfed her small body. This was my first time meeting her in the Breast Cancer Fund offices, the organization she had started years prior. "We become more of the artist than we are, or we become writers, or we decide to make a film, or we start an organization. My way was in kind of an entrepreneurial organization." With the political connections she had made, along with the community of friends in northern California, Andrea had the necessary support. She was dynamic, smart, and quick, the perfect candidate to direct an organization that would be very political and controversial. That was what she wanted — to force people to start thinking, really thinking, about the causes of breast cancer.

A tanned and healthy Andrea told me this story. Petite and energetic, her hair was cut in a practical bob, useful when leading the mountain climbing expeditions hosted by her organization. During those events, Andrea's strident voice carried over snow ridges and steep climbs to guide other women with breast cancer up toward a clear blue sky. By the year I met her, 2000, she had beaten breast cancer.

Soon after activists in Massachusetts had started their work, women like Andrea in the Bay Area began to get concerned about environmental causation. As Brody collected evidence of exposures in women's homes, scientists and activists in California looked inside women's bodies to find chemicals trapped in tissue. Although there is still a limited amount of knowledge about how specific levels of contaminants in the body relate to increases in breast cancer and other diseases, figuring out which chemicals exist offered the possibility of blocking them before they got inside the body. In order to prevent these exposures, California campaigns tie those chemicals to the corporations that produce them. This more radical approach is typical of the "Left coast" and has been, in some ways, more effective.

Women in California turned debates over science into a way to make corporations accountable and our lives safer. Their campaigns are as personal as possible, drawing attention not to what is around us but instead to what is under our skin and in our blood. By moving one step closer, maybe making the most intimate connection between chemicals and breast cancer, California women have leveraged a campaign against makeup companies facilitated by new scientific findings. Political economy followed scientific. Policies came on the footsteps of examining bodies, finding what lay within.

After I met with Andrea that day in San Francisco, I took the elevator down two floors and exited onto Sutter Street. I thought about the breast cancer organizations I had first become acquainted with on the East Coast and now in California. Dwarfed by larger breast cancer organizations and foundations, they had found a point of commonality—taking a preventive approach. They had all also started out at a small kitchen table sharing what they knew and what information they had been unable to find. Some of the women in different locations had met and even worked with one another. But the women in San Francisco seemed more than slightly different. Some were demanding more research, but even more than that, they were attacking corporate interests that make millions and even billions of dollars from breast cancer while being masked by the rhetoric of a cure.

I met Barbara Brenner, the director of Breast Cancer Action, the next day. She had started the other San Francisco–based organization with a national scope. Like Andrea, Barbara was trained as a lawyer. Apart from that, similarities were minimal. She told me how breast cancer activism in the Bay Area had started. Elenore Pred was the first. After her diagnosis, Elenore decided to research what might have caused her illness. She contacted government agencies, doctors, and local organizations but found no real answer. There was almost no information on the causes of the disease, only information about treatment. Frustrated with her search, she invited eleven other women to meet in her living room. They formed what came to be known as Breast Cancer Action. That was 1990. Elenore died the next year.

Brenner had been practicing law for thirteen years before getting breast cancer. That training taught her to speak in sound bites. When asked about her position about any political topic, the responding sentence is generally quotable. When I asked what the purpose of her organization was, she answered simply, "To raise hell." I was not surprised by this answer even though we had met only a few minutes prior. At first, I had interpreted her curt responses to mean that she was annoyed by my simple, graduate student questions. I quickly understood that she does not temper her wit with softness or unnecessary niceties. What you see is what you get. Her appearance is no different. There are no frills, even on fancy occasions. On a day-to-day basis, she sports cropped brown hair, small round glasses and frequently a button-down shirt with jeans. When Breast Cancer Action holds large events, Barbara might switch over to black pants and add a blazer. Her sarcasm and irony persist.

Breast Cancer Action calls itself the "Bad Girls of Breast Cancer." Pins and brochures around the office read, "Think Before You Pink," "Cancer Sucks," and "Prevention First." Perusing their media files shows that Barbara has been quoted in every major publication at least once: the *New York Times*, the *Los Angeles Times*, San Francisco newspapers, and many others. She critiques the overinvestment in mammography, a public focus she believes distracts scientists from finding the cause of the illness. While she knows the scientific literature on breast cancer down to the most recent study, Barbara has been cited in women's magazines, newsweeklies, and public radio, drawing the outline of a larger critique of corporate accountability for a largely unaware public.

"We are a little different from a lot of breast cancer organizations," explained Barbara toward the end of our first meeting. "It's not just about breast cancer. Breast cancer is just a wedge issue." Looking over their organizational documents and the articles in which she was featured, this seemed to be an accurate portrayal. Her organizations ran campaigns against corporate malfeasance and drew attention to conflicts of interest in government agencies. These widely publicized projects gave Breast Cancer Action national attention.

I left Brenner's office on the third floor of a brick building in downtown San Francisco and walked down Market Street to the bay. Looking out over the wind-whipped water, a gray ocean stretched out in front of me. It was like the one I had woken up to on arriving at Port Jefferson, Long Island, but this time it was the Pacific instead of the Atlantic. Only white bobbing boats interrupted the view. As I reflected on my meeting with Barbara and Andrea and reviewed my materials for other interviews in the Bay Area, I began to realize that the women on this coast were extreme and uncompromising, creative in their approach.

Elenore Pred and Andrea Martin had started their organizations because more and more women in the Bay Area seemed to be getting breast cancer. At that point, scientists had yet to show it, but they saw illness spreading like mold in a seaside home, quiet, stealthy, and uncontrollable. Scientists in the Bay Area had in fact been calculating cancer rates, but they had yet to be widely publicized before 1994. "People in the area were shocked when we released the study," said Bob Hiatt, former director of a division of the Northern California Cancer Registry. "I guess we shouldn't have been surprised considering the headlines read, 'Breast Cancer Rates Highest in the World.'"

The registry had found that some counties in the Bay Area had the highest rates of breast cancer scientists had ever seen. Marin County, just north of the city, was the worst. Shock pervaded the community. Phones began ringing at the Cancer Registry. Questions and assertions about the reason for heightened rates were raised. Experts gave the typical response—diet, higher levels of education, later childbirth, wealth, and birth control usage.

Francine Levien, a Marin resident, was concerned about other factors that could be at play—the munitions dumped in the bay in the 1960s, pesticides sprayed on the beautifully landscaped lawns in Marin, and the vast range of exposures traced back to the environment. In 1995, one year after the Massachusetts Breast Cancer Coalition got funding for the Silent Spring Institute and the Northern California Cancer Center released its report, Levien brought local women together at her kitchen table to found Marin Breast Cancer Watch. She was close to seventy at that point, energetic and sharp witted despite her advanced years and seemingly delicate body.

The women in that area are well educated and wealthy. In fact, Marin County is known for its affluence. It is more lush and less concrete than San Francisco, and that difference can be felt in the people, whose countenance seem more delicate. The houses are mammoth. They rise up out of skillfully landscaped yards or hang off the side of sharply rising hills. All seem to overlook the ocean with a sense of consequence and ease.

"We have got to look at environmental issues," Francine said to her new board stubbornly. "We have an epidemic on our hands in Marin. The report said that we have the highest rates in the world. Why? There has got to be something in the environment." Breast cancer rates in Marin County are extreme, 40 percent higher than the rest of the United States. Once the community heard that, ex-hippy radicals who had turned Marin into a post-1960s haven started to push for research into what was causing the high rates. But environmental causes were not at the top of their list. In fact, no one had thought of it yet, and Francine was being more progressive than even her radical colleagues appreciated.

The board flatly returned Francine's gaze. They were wary of this kind of approach. Sure, there were a lot of environmentalists in Marin, but there were also a lot of conservative interests, businessmen and women, Republicans. They would not support an organization with political tendencies like Francine's. "You know what a lot of people around here are like," responded one board member hesitantly. "This may not be the way to go."

"Look, when I got breast cancer, doctors told me I should do what everyone else was doing. They wanted me to have surgery and radiation, and I just said good-bye. Everyone was sure I would be dead soon." She paused. Her gentle eyes, framed by soft wrinkles and a halo of short white hair, were intent. "I put myself on a very strict macrobiotic diet, then I went to see a macrobiotic counselor, and he put me on a even stricter diet. I carried my food with me wherever I went, and I really stayed for one year, absolutely fine. Brown rice every day, lots of vegetables, seaweed, the whole nine yards." She told her own story of breast cancer—how she had waited to get an appointment with the Dali Lama's doctor, whose office was close by, but with no luck, Francine gave in to a mastectomy. Her lump had grown large enough to press on her rib cage and felt uncomfortable. Friends were scared that she had not taken a traditional treatment routine. "I had to give up on that. This, I can't give up on," she finished, refusing to budge.

Mary Gould, another board member who had been diagnosed with breast cancer and was fighting a losing battle, agreed. She argued that something had to be done to prevent other women from going through the same hell. The board gave in, at least partly, and began to bring in speakers from around the country. At the same time, Francine contacted Lorraine Pace, the original mapper on Long Island. She was now an expert on how local women could figure out patterns of breast cancer in their area. Francine wanted to know what Marin's patterns were. The scientists from the Northern California Cancer Center who had generated the statistics had not looked at the geographic distribution. Only those patterns could help specify if there were local sources of exposure around which cancer clusters grouped. Francine could not think of anything in particular but refused to buy the idea that women were getting sick just because they were wealthy and well educated and postponed having kids.

MAKING PAIN PUBLIC

When Francine started her organization, she talked to the other organization directors like Andrea. At that point, in the mid-1990s, Martin was heading up a new project maybe more controversial than Levien's. A few years prior, *Time* magazine had published the photographs of Matuschka, a woman with a single mastectomy who had taken portraits of herself nude from the waist up. She was beautiful—thin, with a cropped head of black hair—striking. The black-and-white image captured the crags and crevices left in place of her right breast. The title ran, "You can't look away anymore." Matuschka's photograph portrayed the physical outcome of breast cancer to the public, which was accustomed to images of patched-up survivors with their families, hiding the real damage of the disease.

Martin was inspired by Matuschka. She developed a new campaign that, in her words, "forces us to acknowledge that we are being subjected to a deadly and disfiguring epidemic directed at our culture's most profound symbol of sexuality and nurture. They also help us understand that a true appreciation of breasts requires us to act more responsibly in the way we treat women, their bodies, and the disease" (Martin 2000). A series of posters and billboards of young women with mastectomies nude from the waist up, similar to Matuschka's photograph, went up around the Bay Area. The images were of models who typified beauty—thin, young, white—with Andrea's mastectomy scars digitally drawn onto the photograph.

The Obsessed with Breasts campaign drew criticism. San Francisco residents received these billboards with shock, admiration, and dismay. Some activists worried that the ads would scare women from seeing their doctors and create an unrealistic image of the disease as striking only young, thin, white women. Cartoons from the *San Francisco Chronicle* and the *San Francisco Examiner* and news sources all over the United States and Europe also covered the story.

In its announcement of the campaign, the Breast Cancer Fund addressed the criticisms it knew would be leveraged, foremost being that people did not want to see the ravages of the disease. It likened the campaign to the movie *Saving Private Ryan*, which claimed to reveal the realities of war. Film critics not only excused but also supported the graphic portrayal of thousands of deaths meant to make viewers think twice about the ravages of war. The Breast Cancer Fund's campaign pamphlet claimed that the billboards were meant to "lift the polite veil separating these images from breast cancer . . . and brings us in touch with the very real consequences of the disease."

WHAT IS IN YOUR BODY?

While some groups were drawing attention to the ravages of breast cancer on the outside of the body, others began to investigate what on the inside had been the cause. While groups on the East Coast pulled together money for highly controversial science, it took some time before California activists did the same. By the late 1990s, Andrea and Francine had either initiated or participated in new research that took a closer look at what could be causing the disease. Like the East Coasters, the work was highly charged both politically and scientifically. But the West Coast women pushed the envelope even further, taking it beyond science to action.

Andrea Martin's work brought her recognition outside the breast cancer community. Bay Area elites and national leaders knew about her. The

Environmental Working Group (EWG), an environmental watchdog organization in Washington, D.C., had heard of her. In 2003, EWG and the Mount Sinai School of Medicine, with another environmental organization, Commonweal, tested the blood of nine celebrities, including Andrea, investigative reporter Bill Moyers, and executive director of Health Care Without Harm Charlotte Brody.

"Around that time, we began to notice that chemicals in makeup were starting to show up in the blood of humans," said Jane Houlihan, the assistant director of research at EWG. Jane's team took blood and urine samples to measure the celebrities' body burden of chemicals. Body burden studies, also called biomonitoring, evaluate the amount of chemicals in an individual's blood, urine, breast milk, or tissue. While these studies cannot tell scientists what chemicals cause any particular disease, they provide information on what is currently stored in our bodies.

The EWG researchers came up with startling and disturbing findings. All the individuals they tested had chemicals in their blood. It was just a matter of which ones and how much. After testing for 214 possible compounds, the researchers found lead, mercury, arsenic, polychlorinated biphenyls, dioxins, and a range of other chemicals that cause birth defects, cancer, reproductive problems, and other health issues. Seventy-six of the chemicals they tested for cause cancer, and ninety-four are linked to neurological development problems. Andrea Martin had 101 of the possible 214 in her blood. Although that seems like an extraordinary amount, another participant, Bill Moyers, had eighty-seven chemicals in his body. Other participants had similar levels.

Soon after, her picture appeared in the *New York Times* with the caption, "Warning—Andrea Martin's blood contains 59 cancer causing industrial chemicals." Andrea was quoted in the accompanying article as saying, "My body is a record of the environmental history of my life." Around the same time, the Centers for Disease Control and Prevention (CDC 2003) also issued its report card on America's chemical body burden; 2,500 donors were tested, and the CDC concluded that chemical residues have polluted most Americans, including lead, cadmium, pesticides, and a slew of other products, all associated with different kinds of health effects.

While that biomonitoring study relied on blood, others have used breast milk. Scientists have begun to wonder how chemicals in the breast might be linked to breast cancer. Breast milk is replete with toxins. It contains such a high level of contaminants that the Food and Drug Administration (FDA) would never put it on the grocery store shelf (Environmental Protection Agency 2000). Toxins accumulate in the breast because they store in fatty tissue, like that in the breast. It is possible that this concentration of toxics plays a role in the disease. Scientists are also using other bodily fluids to link chemicals to breast cancer risk.

Dale Sandler, chief of the Epidemiology Branch at the National Institute of Environmental Health Sciences (NIEHS), began testing this hypothesis with what is called the Sister Study in 2002. She and her colleague, Clarice Weinberg, chief of the NIEHS Biostatistics Branch, direct one of the largest federal studies of what environmental factors might cause breast cancer. Both Sandler and Weinberg are following 25,000 pairs of sisters from four states where one has had the disease and the other has not. They began looking for volunteers by visiting the Race for the Cure sites in Providence, Rhode Island; Tucson, Arizona; Tampa, Florida; and St. Louis, Missouri. In 2012, the researchers will stop examining the daily behaviors of the sisters and try to answer their most important questions: are the causes genetic, diet, early menstruation, a household or environmental chemical, or a gene–environment interaction?

At that point, Sandler and Weinberg will have amassed ten years' worth of blood, urine samples, and toenail clippings — all biomonitoring data — and annual surveys of daily behavior. The Sister Study is the first long-term research project on breast cancer that collects detailed information about environmental exposures. Its recruiting method may also signify the first occasion on which the environment became a serious issue at Race for the Cure.

While American researchers have just begun to use biomonitoring studies, European countries are particularly keen on the technique since Swedish researchers found flame retardants in breast milk in the late 1990s (Meironyte et al. 1999). Since then, some European countries annually screen for chemicals. Bans on these chemicals have since been issued. Governments in North America have been slower to regulate them. Possibly as a result, researchers have recently found that levels of flame retardants in breast milk are much higher for American women (EWG report). This is particularly true of California residents. In 2002, a group of breast cancer and environmental activists in California created an action plan to reduce exposures to chemicals and pushed for biomonitoring as one way to do so. The Environmental Protection Agency of California took the hint and initiated its own biomonitoring study.

Finding chemicals in individual's blood, urine, or milk is more than scary. It is damning. Chemicals can be present, even though a person had no knowledge he or she ever consumed or was exposed to them. Presence of a chemical in your body makes two things clear. First, there was at least that much to start out with and probably more. Many chemicals seep out of the body over time. Second, something has to be done to make sure that does not happen to others. No one argues that a chemical inside a person is a good thing. Social action is almost inherent in biomonitoring. When debate ceases about whether we are exposed to something, more science is mandated to figure out what those exposures—those chemicals in our bodies—might be doing. Biomonitoring seems like a simple invention, but it has massive scientific and regulatory ramifications. The California women knew how to use science to make a point, and they had made it.

But while science, like biomonitoring, moves on slowly and incrementally, the leaders of the movement who made the science happen passed away. On August 6, 2001, Andrea Martin died from brain cancer. Her breast cancer had begun in 1988, and it moved to her brain in 2001. Her daughter and husband were devastated. The breast cancer community felt the loss acutely. Andrea had been one of the most outspoken leaders for innovative approaches to the illness. Her role had not been to provide services or make arguments about the need for treatments. Instead, she had pushed the community to think that it was a political illness. Like the radical activism of her area, she had made many public stinks. Francine also died that same year of a recurrence. Andrea's and Francine's deaths marked a new period in breast cancer activism in the Bay Area.

KILLING YOUR CLIENT

While the scientists at NIEHS and EWG collected data and deciphered which chemicals were getting into the blood, Barbara Brenner, Deb Forter, and a smattering of local organizations across the country started Follow the Money to make corporate fund-raisers for breast cancer accountable. This fight soon led them to a new battleground: ingredients lists in personal care products. The coalition has drawn attention to a little-known fact about personal care products—that the government does not regulate their ingredients. The FDA (1995) admits that "a cosmetic manufacturer may use almost any raw material as a cosmetic ingredient and market the product without an approval from FDA." The agency is woefully unable or unwilling to monitor and protect us from these substances. Instead, the FDA allows the Cosmetics Review Board to regulate its own production practices. In fact, while the FDA is meant to oversee the board, in reality one nonvoting member of the FDA is a part of the Review Board, and there is little accountability to the FDA. Put in place in the early 1970s, the Cosmetics Board has approved the vast majority of proposed ingredients to be passed (Schapiro 2005). According to Jane Houlihan of EWG, 89 percent of the 10,500 ingredients in personal care products have not being evaluated for safety. Many of these products contain known carcinogens. Fifty-five percent of products contain a penetration enhancer that enables the product to be more easily absorbed in the bloodstream. Officials on the board are industry representatives who have entrenched interested in the board's policies. Making cosmetics safer will probably never come from the board itself or from the FDA. The coalition arose to address this gap.

One of the coalition's first questions centered on products used to raise breast cancer awareness. Some include chemicals with fairly well proven carcinogenicity (Ardies and Dees 1998; Damstra et al. 2002). For example, Avon raises funds for breast cancer through its Cosmetics for the Cure and Kiss Breast Cancer Good-Bye cause-marketing campaigns. Proceeds from these promotions contribute to the company's $350 million global total for fundraising as of 2004. Ironically, one of the products that Avon sells for its campaign is laden with potentially carcinogenic chemicals. Avon Kiss Goodbye to Breast Cancer Brilliant Moisture Lipcolor is in a thin pink tube and comes in several colors: Crusade Rose, Determined Red, Cherub Cheer, Courageous Coral, Brave Brocade, and Spice of Life. Avon's advertising claims that "every lipstick will come with the free Avon Crusade 'Guide to Better Breast Health,' which provides vital information on breast cancer, early detection, medical and support resources, and a glossary of terms." It costs four dollars, and half the proceeds go to the Avon Foundation's programs for breast cancer.

EWG created a detailed list of the ingredients of these lipsticks. They concluded that each lip color contains six ingredients linked to cancer or another illness, one ingredient linked to immune or nervous system toxicity, and several others that may cause an immune system response like itching or burning (EWG 2008). Four ingredients in the lipstick bioaccumulate in the body, meaning that when a biomonitoring study is done, the chemicals will show up in blood, tissue, or urine. Thirty-seven ingredients are being used in the lipstick even though they have never been studied for their effects on human health. This Brilliant Moisture Lipcolor might even be illegal in Europe since one of its ingredients cannot be used there, except under certain conditions.

The EWG database has also shown that another product, Avon Breast Cancer Crusade Limited-Edition Celebrity Crusade Nailwear Nail Enamel, may be slightly less harmful but still contains ingredients you would not want soaking into your body. Most nail polishes contain phthalates, which are plasticizers that make nail polish pliable and nonbrittle but that cause cancer. This nail polish does not. However, like the lip color, there are a number of chemicals that have not been tested, that may cause an adverse immune system response, or that are toxic to the liver (EWG 2008). More threatening yet, butyl acetate is the second ingredient on the list. It is linked to infertility or being unable to have a healthy, full-term pregnancy (Correa et al. 1996). Other ingredients in the nail polish are being studied but might harm health in additional ways.

Avon is not the only breast cancer fund-raiser whose agenda does not match its profit mandate. Estée Lauder initiated one of the largest breast cancer funding organizations, the Breast Cancer Research Foundation. But the company also has suspect chemicals in some products, like one promoting anti-aging effects that contains methylparaben, butylparaben, polyparaben, and isobutylparaben, ingredients that have been linked to cancer because of their estrogenic activity (Pedersen et al. 2000; Routledge et al. 1998) even in the seemingly small amounts we encounter every day (Oishi 2002). Other problematic ingredients include endocrine-disrupting chemicals and products with reproductive toxicity.

The Follow the Money Coalition first investigated the destination of funds raised through Avon's breast cancer walks and was successful in getting Avon to be more efficient with the dollars it raised. Their second step was to get shareholders to vote that certain, suspect ingredients in makeup be studied better. In a *New York Times* ad, Breast Cancer Action wrote, "Philanthropy or Hypocrisy?" The text described the carcinogenic chemicals in makeup made by companies that raised millions in funds for breast cancer. Coalition members, like Breast Cancer Action, collaborated with two asset management companies, Walden Asset Management and Trillium Asset Management, and two mutual funds, Domini Social Investments and the Women's Equity Fund, in order to buy the sufficient number of stocks to be allowed to attend shareholder meetings and try to influence manufacturing. Although they never owned a significant number of shares, they had enough to get in the door.

Leading the way for the group, Deb began the discussion by faxing a letter to the senior vice president of Avon, Gilbert Klemann II: "The Massachusetts Breast Cancer Coalition is submitting for inclusion in the next proxy statement, in accordance with Rule 14a-8 of these General Rules, the enclosed shareholder proposal. The proposal asks our company to produce a report to shareholders evaluating the feasibility of removing dibutyl phthalates from Avon Products." Phthalates are a controversial ingredient in personal care products. They are particularly common in nail polish and are used to make skin moisturizer soft. They cannot be found in the ingredients list of most products because the FDA does not mandate their inclusion.

Methyl and ethylparaben are equally controversial, but more often they appear at the end of the ingredients list in most shampoos and lotions. Some Avon products also contain these chemicals. Scientists have known the dangers of phthalates and the paraben family of chemicals for some time (Colborn et al. 2003). They are carcinogenic. Animal studies showed that male reproductive organs are damaged by exposure, and normal hormonal balance in utero is also disturbed.

Deb found it ironic that Avon was raising millions of dollars for breast cancer but at the same time was producing a product that could harm the very people it meant to help. She was willing to give them the benefit of the doubt and help them tackle the administrative monster of taking phthalates out of their cosmetics. The report she attached to the letter was long and detailed. It stated the most basic facts at the top. Four shades of Avon nail polish—Speed Dry Top Shine, Tough Enough Base Coat, and On the Mend Nail Mender—contained dibutyl phthalate (DBP). Almost six months previously, the Department of Health and Human Services had reviewed animal studies showing that the chemicals reduced fertility and fouled up the growth of male reproductive organs (Colborn et al. 2002). Baby birds exposed to it in the wild were born with multiple legs. The same was true for alligators. Fish became deformed.

The Centers for Disease Control is increasingly concerned about these exposures. By its estimates, more than 3 million women of childbearing age were exposed to DBP, over twenty times more than other people (Houlihan et al. 2002). This meant that they are way out of the safe range for birth defects. The defects in humans are like those in animals. Human babies don't have extra arms or legs, but, like the alligators, frogs and birds, their development in the womb could be disrupted, causing problems after birth.

American researchers are just a small part of the scientific community that has been studying what happens when humans are exposed to these chemicals. Other countries tend to take these threats more seriously, creating councils and scientific calls to action. In the period of time that Deb and Barbara were waiting to hear back from Avon, the Canadian government issued a call to action on research connecting health and the environment. "The key research themes and priorities in Canada include: outdoor and workplace environments; water and air quality; toxic substances, meals, and endocrine disrupting substances; respiratory health and cancer," it reported. "These issues are similar to the priorities of international organizations and other countries" (Canadian Institute of Health Research 2002, 3).

Soon after, the European Union issued a comparable statement. "Europe's citizens are concerned about the potential impact of the environment on their health and expect policy makers to act," it read. "As individuals we can make certain choices about our lifestyles which affect our health, but we also rely on public authorities to provide us with reliable information on which to base our decisions" (Commission of European Communities 2004, 3). The statement continued, "We cannot select the quality of air that we breathe or always protect ourselves from exposure to pollutants that may build up in our bodies—sometimes even before we are born." In an attempt to prevent as many exposures as possible, the European Union had begun instituting regulatory measures in 2001 aimed at substances that had not been tested adequately for their impacts on human health. But this document implied that the policies needed to be applied more strongly. In order to do that, government officials were in the process of developing a plan to ban carcinogenic materials from makeup.

Six months after Deb faxed the letter, the shareholders meeting was approaching. Gil Klemann, vice president of Avon Products, responded to her letter and disputed the statements about parabens. Klemann submitted a counterargument and had submitted it to the Avon's Shareholder Advocacy Association. In his letter, Klemann argued that the Cosmetic Ingredient Review Expert Panel had reviewed the science investigating parabens and decided that the group of chemicals was safe. He claimed that the panel was an independent body of experts that was reliable and had no investment in keeping parabens in the makeup. In fact, the Cosmetic, Toiletry and Fragrance Association funded the panel. This meant that it was not the best judge of the safeness of parabens. It had a vested interest in keeping the ingredients as they were. This would save cosmetic companies the hassle and expense of needing to change production practices and find a safer alternative—sort of the fox guarding the henhouse.

Klemann also stated that many studies had addressed the issue of carcinogenicity and had come out with approval for the use of parabens. But the few studies he focused on were from 1968 and 1974, pre-dating the discovery that parabens are harmful (Domini Social Investments LLC, letter to Edward Smith, Esq., regarding Avon products, 2003). Deb's letter pointed this out, along with the Cosmetic Ingredient Review Expert Panel's conflict of interest.

Adam Kanzer and Kimberly Gladman, the heads of the Shareholder Advocacy Association, defended Deb's letter. "Dear Gil," they wrote, "Thank you for your letter in opposition to our proposal. However, we believe that the statement contains false and misleading statements. We request that these sentences be removed." Kanzer and Gladman picked out parts of Klemann's argument that were opaque to shareholders who did not have a background in chemistry and other arguments that were distinctly false.

Navigating the administration and paperwork of making a shareholders request was new to Deb and Barbara. But nonetheless, they had successfully introduced a proposal that would be voted on at the annual meeting. At minimum, they wanted to get the ingredients reviewed by the company. They were allowed to attend the shareholders meeting and testify in support of their proposal. That year's meeting was in the W Hotel in New York City.

Deb took the train down from Boston. From across the street, all she could see was a set of two-tone flags hanging from the front of the building. Scaffolding rigged for construction on the face of the thirty-story building above disguised the entrance. The street was bustling in that part of town. At 51st Street, she was close enough to the heart of midtown to feel the pulse of Manhattan.

It was March and still cold in New York. She ducked out of the wind and pushed through the rotating glass door edged with gold entering the marble-floored lobby. Security guards wearing black T-shirts, slacks, and dark sunglasses and slicked hair stood in pairs around the room. They almost looked like patrons with their casual air and nonchalant chatting. They glanced at Deb. Clearly she was no threat. Deb met Barbara Brenner and several other women from the coalition in the lobby. They walked up the curved staircase, signed in, and found a seat in the meeting room.

After watching the presentations about Avon's financial standing and new products, they made their statements. The board responded superficially and dismissively, although the public shareholders attending the meeting applauded their statements. The proposition of studying the possibility of removing phthalates and other chemicals from makeup made it to the proxy statement, and votes in favor had reached 3 percent. While it was not high enough to get it adopted by the board, it was enough of a vote in favor to allow it to be brought up again at the following shareholders meeting. The small group of advocates felt vindicated by achieving this benchmark and had definitely made an impact on the executives at the Avon Corporation. Yet taking it a step further to protect women was impossible. Most countries that the company sells to do not legislate against these ingredients, so there was no regulation for the company to comply with.

But the group kept on the issue, continuing to submit proposals to Avon and appear at shareholders meetings. In 2004, things took a turn for the better. Soon after the meeting, later that year, the European Union decided that a certain set of 110 ingredients could not be included in imported products. This meant that Avon had to change how it manufactured European makeup. The company would have to remove phthalates from its products for the European market by September 11, 2004.

Shelley Alpern from Trillium Investments had been working with Deb and Barbara on the resolution when she heard from an old roommate that the company was not happy about it and did not agree with the European Union's scientific basis. It reported to the Investor Responsibility Research Center that "the European ban on DBP was not based on a specific risk assessment for cosmetic products. In contrast, the Cosmetic Ingredient Review (CIR), an independent, nonprofit scientific body that is recognized by the FDA and publishes its findings in a peer reviewed journal, recently reaffirmed its position that DBP may be used safely in cosmetics products."

Battles over the independence of the scientists at CIR had already been fought. The more important point was whether Avon would remove the chemicals from its American products. It was promising to do feasibility studies and possibly remove the nail products with DBP from the market. The only pressure to do this came from other companies, such as Aveda and Osea, which were already doing it, and from the activists. No one else seemed to know about the ingredients, and no one in the United States would be monitoring the ingredients.

There has been little government action in the United States following the EU model. The federal government ignored the new EU policies. But certain states attempted to adopt similar policies. California was the first state. The first bill followed on the heels of the EU proposal, but legislators killed it. In early 2005, Judi Chu, a representative from Monterey Park, California, proposed a compromise. Rather than the broad range of chemicals covered by the European Union, her bill would strike carcinogenic ingredients in cosmetics. In June, Senator Carole Migden from San Francisco followed it with a bill to the California legislature requiring cosmetic manufacturers to report the ingredients of their products that might cause cancer or birth defects. This bill would at least mandate that manufacturers provide an online list of the ingredients. This legislation, SB484, was passed with an eight-to-four vote. Governor Schwarzenegger still had to approve it, although he was not taking a stance on it yet (Gledhill 2005). California was the only state radical enough to adopt this measure. Federal agencies made no advances.

After pressure and changes in EU policy, Avon decided to take a baby step toward safer products and removed DBP from its products on the American market—one small step for a company and possibly a giant leap for womankind.

Robin had gotten well enough to begin the process of reconstruction. This meant the tissue expanders put under her skin during the mastectomy would be replaced by implants. Many women undergo this procedure. Robin's experience was harder than some. Her rounds of chemo were followed by rounds of antibiotics to get rid of several infections. One of these bouts returned her to the hospital for close to a week.

Bed rest was accompanied by twinges that wrapped around her chest and back. The pain made it hard to function normally, taking the kids to school and keeping the household running. Doctors' bills were coming in. Even though most of the procedures were covered by insurance, some fell on the family's shoulders. Money was tight, and Eddy was stressed.

I went to see her. She made no pretense for me or for the camera I brought. She wore an oversized red sweatshirt and baggy pants. Circles ran under her eyes, and the dark roots of her long blond hair had grown to several inches in length. "I am doing everything I can to get better," she said to me, sitting on a stool in the kitchen. The kids were at school, and the house was quiet. "So much has been going on. My mom got sick. Little Eddy got bitten by a dog. We have been trying to renovate the house, but with all these bills, it is just too much."

Stress was evident in her face. Creases wrapped around her mouth and ran across her forehead. She frowned. "I am taking the Tamoxifen now," she said. "I will take it for five years. I don't know if it is just me, but there are so many side effects." She pulled the miniature pamphlet out that accompanied the bottle of pills and unfolded it. "Dizziness, blurred vision, bleeding, rash, there are so many. I just feel like I have them all. I want to know when all of this is going to end."

III

SECTION III

Chapter Seven

The Way Out

The first law of ecology is that everything is related to everything else.

—Barry Commoner

Two years before I finished graduate school, my mother was diagnosed with a rare lung infection—non-HIV mycobacterium avium complex. It was something I had never heard of. She had started coughing, then finding blood next to her pillow in the morning. The doctor said it was increasingly common although still in small numbers, especially among "older women in the South." I tried to guess what might be special about these women—what they were doing more or exposed to more often—but couldn't. I was on a trip in South America doing research for my dissertation at the time. My mom and I were communicating mainly by e-mail. Phone calls were almost a dollar per minute. At first, I did not realize how serious it was. No matter how specific an e-mail is, gravity is erased. Eventually when we spoke, it became clear to me. It was potentially terminal. A bit like cancer, she would have to take regimens of pills to get rid of the illness, mainly powerful antibiotics that might destroy her liver, eyesight, and heart. I was meant to be in Brazil for another few months. She told me to not worry and to stay there. Sitting in a small apartment in Rio de Janeiro looking out over pointed city hilltops, thousands of miles and an expanse of ocean away, I felt paralyzed.

Taking graduate courses on environmental health had already reminded me of what happened so long ago on Bishop Lake. I wondered about this rare lung infection and if it was linked to what happened to my family decades ago. I had already begun to be more aware of the things I was exposed to. Certain types of lotions and shampoos were no longer on my shopping list. I no longer wore nail polish despite inheriting stubby, pudgy fingers from my father's side of the family that needed prettying up. After several years of reading endless papers about toxins I came into contact with daily, I had not become paranoid but very careful. I looked at ingredients lists before purchasing products. My refrigerator was full of mainly organic food. More often than before, I wrote letters or e-mails to my state representatives about regulations under consideration. These began to be my very small steps toward making my world safe. I know these are important measures, and if taken by enough people, they will radically change what is available in the grocery store, the cost of safer products, and the production practices of manufacturers and farmers.

In the states of New York, Massachusetts, and California, things have already begun to change to one degree or another. Karen Miller's work, along with activists all over Long Island, has led to local ordinances that alert communities to chemical spraying. At minimum, mothers can keep their toddlers from running onto a lawn glistening with pesticides, and golfers can wait until the chemicals have penetrated the soil before they play a round. In some areas, women like Barbara Balaban have even convinced county governments that there are safe alternatives to pesticides. Massachusetts has developed the Toxics Use Reduction Institute, which helps businesses figure out how to replace chemicals that are harmful to health. The Alliance for a Healthy Tomorrow is also close to achieving passage of the Act for a Healthy Massachusetts. It would add more support for replacing toxic chemicals and evaluating which ones need to be destroyed next.

California is by far the most forward thinking state in our country. Several cities in the Bay Area, including Berkeley and Oakland, have passed precautionary principle ordinances that encourage governments to buy nontoxic products, and the state itself has angered industry in its attempt to track toxins better. In 2005, legislators passed the California Safe Cosmetics Act, which forced manufacturers to supply information about toxic ingredients, like phthalates, that are in their products. Barbara Brenner helped by cosponsoring the bill. In other states, consumers apply lotions and other products to their bodies without fully knowing what the ingredients are. A law for a state as big as California may correct that.

These are beginning changes. Other measures are necessary if we are to understand what toxic exposures are doing to public health and if we truly want to slow rising rates of cancer. Making cancer an anomaly rather than normal will take political pressure, time, and specific action. First, we must keep track of illness trends to have evidence that change is needed. Second, we must slow the production of potentially toxic chemicals. They are as dangerous as arms proliferation, simply more subtle and insidious. Finally, the way we make things has to change. This means addressing the very basics of manufacturing. We must change the industrial assumption that making toxics is acceptable.

HAMSTRINGING OUR HEALTH

By June 11, 2001, it was the beginning of summer at Adelphi University in Garden City, New Jersey. Even so, first thing in the morning, the ballroom in the Student Center was full, ready for a Senate hearing on environmental contamination and disease clusters. Three senators—Lincoln Chafee from Rhode Island, Hillary Clinton from New York, and Harry Reid of Nevada—were present. Following their initial statements, five state congresspersons gave testimony. Scientists had also come to testify. Phil Landrigan from Mount Sinai Medical Center; Merilee Gammon, the lead scientist on the Long Island Breast Cancer Study Project; and Dr. Lynn Goldman of the Johns Hopkins were there. This was one of about seventy other kinds of Senate-held hearings during the rest of the year. In this one, a debate would be held about how to move forward on environmental risks and improve health.

Senators Reid and Clinton already favored investigating environmental links to cancer. They needed more support to get the funding for a nationwide system that would track where cases of illness arose. These data could then be compared to environmental exposures in any area. Two months earlier, the senators had introduced Senate Bill 830, the Breast Cancer and Environmental Research Act. With Clinton's and others' support, they hoped to gain more than $150 million to study environmental causes of breast cancer.

"A study recently conducted in Sweden showed that environmental factors may matter more than genetics in determining whether a woman is diagnosed with breast cancer," reported Chafee. "This study found that the environment—what we eat, breathe, drink, and smoke, including how we live and which chemicals we are exposed to—accounts for roughly twice the risk of cancer than genes do.

"There is a reason so many women in Long Island are being diagnosed with breast cancer, and I believe that the environment here holds the key to this mystery." Chafee finished, and moved on to allow the scientists to testify (Senate Environment and Public Works Committee Field Hearing 2001).

Goldman was trained in both medicine and public health. She was a professor at the best school of public health in the world. Being at Johns Hopkins meant that someone should listen when you testify. This time it was a Senate committee.

"Who is guarding our health?" she asked the audience. "The answer is that the public health service has fallen short of its duty—lacking the tracking, troops, and leadership. This is exactly where our federal government is needed—to develop the tracking and monitoring systems, supply the troops, and offer the leadership to prevent chronic disease." Like the other scientists there, she knew that the hearing's topic was important not just to the advancement of knowledge but also to the people affected by chronic diseases like breast cancer. Long Island women testified about their frustrated attempts to find out about breast cancer rates in their area and how they had been forced to instigate new studies to fill in missing data. Goldman had years of experience with clusters like the ones on Long Island. She had investigated childhood cancer clusters in response to some of the 1,000 requests made by concerned communities around the country. The National Academy of Sciences was estimating that 25 percent of developmental diseases increasing in children, like cerebral palsy, autism, and mental retardation, were caused by environmental factors. But tracking these illnesses was the only way to figure out if there were local environmental factors increasing rates.

She related to the committee how health tracking had led to the eradication of polio, yellow fever, and typhoid, illnesses that Americans now longer thought about twice. But that kind of system was no longer in place. "We never modernized our public health system to respond to today's health threats. As a result, we are hamstringing our health specialists from finding solutions and effectively taking action—regardless of whether it's childhood cancer or a nationwide asthma epidemic."

Goldman, Landrigan, and the others testifying for the tracking system were thinking about public rather than individual causes of disease. Their approach meant observing human responses to contaminants in the air, food, and water—seeing how populations in geographic areas developed illness. This was very different than the biomedical model used by many researchers. Two hundred years ago, when John Snow broke the handle off a water pump that spouted cholera-infested water into community hands (Fine 2004), the general public believed deeply in the environment being a carrier of disease. Things had changed a lot since then.

We have largely left that model of disease prevention behind and are headed farther away from it. Even the governmental agency charged with connecting environment to public health, the National Institute of Environmental Health Science, is putting an increasing number of research dollars into genetic research or studying the individual as separate from the social and environmental context in which he or she lives (Department of Health and Human Services 2007). While this may result in more targeted treatments for individuals who have access to health care, it leaves most of the world helpless to prevent disease. As the World Health Organization (2003) states, "Molecular genome research will reveal a tremendous amount of information on cancer but it is not clear how easy these discoveries will translate into *actual lives saved* and may well be restricted to rare cancers" (emphasis added). With the growing number and type of illnesses caused by environment, this research trajectory may lead to a public health catastrophe.

POLITICS OR ECONOMY?

Before chlordane was banned and before it was sprayed inside my childhood home, manufacturers amassed millions of dollars from selling the chemical. Like the profits from that single chemical, billions of dollars are made from other cancer-causing chemicals or products every year. Possibly the biggest of these markets is oil. Polycyclic aromatic hydrocarbons (PAHs) are released when oil is burned in the combustion process in a car, truck, factory, or any other engine that uses fuel. They have contributed to the rise of lung cancers, asthma, heart disease, and probably many other illnesses, including breast cancer. One of the studies on Long Island found that women with 50 percent more PAH in their blood had a 25 percent increase in breast cancer risk (Gammon et al. 2002a).

The lives lost to these diseases are not counted in the high prices of gasoline that we are charged at the pump. The consumer does not pay, nor do the companies making astronomical profits from oil sales every year. As Michael Dorsey, a professor of environmental studies at Dartmouth College, says, "In the quarter ended December 31, 2005, ExxonMobil announced it earned $10.7 billion—$115 million a day for each of the ninety-two days of the quarter, $5 million each hour, or more than $80,000 every minute and almost $1,350 per second of that quarter" (personal communication 2007). Every hour that Chevron makes $5 million, we lose five women to breast cancer. The oil industry lobbies the American government to the tune of millions per year. As we have learned from the presidency of George W. Bush, government is often in the oil industry's palm. This means lives lost.

The veiled connections between the industries that expose our families to hazards and the politicians who make decisions about regulating those exposures make it difficult to tell which is the real obstacle to changing national practices—economics or politics. A more relevant question might be why both our economic leaders and government representatives don't make public health more of a priority. They themselves, as well as their daughters and sons, will lose years of their lives to cancers and other diseases caused by the very sales and contributions that put money in their pockets.

Although he was referring to a different system of oppression than the one making us sick with cancers and physical illness, Martin Luther King Jr.'s plea to change injustice, so aptly argued almost half a century ago, is still relevant today. He said,

> This is where we are. Where do we go from here? First, we must massively assert our dignity and worth. We must stand up amidst a system that still oppresses us and develop an unassailable and majestic sense of values.

There are many groups today addressing the injustice that all people in the world must be exposed to toxics in order to benefit the few. Breast cancer is not the only disease caused by toxics in the environment. There is a laundry list of others linked to the very same chemicals associated with breast cancer risk. They have similarly freakishly high rates or are headed quickly in that direction. Endocrine disruptors and other chemicals that are proving to increase breast cancer risk also cause many other illnesses. For example, the recent, dramatic rise in prostate cancer may have analogous roots. In 2007, an estimated 218,890 men were diagnosed with prostate cancer. So similar are biological mechanisms in causing breast and prostate cancers that treatment regimens overlap. AstraZeneca's largest product, Zoladex, is a hormone used to treat both breast and prostate cancers. And so there is financial gain to be had from a range of illnesses. In 2007, there were around 52,170 cases of uterine cancer and 22,430 women with ovarian cancer (American Cancer Society 2007). Stunted neurological development in children is blossoming around the country in the form of autism and attention deficit disorder. Children's cancers are also on the rise.

Possibly the most troubling of these illnesses are those that affect children. It is becoming increasingly apparent that children are much more vulnerable to the pesticides we spray on our lawns or the cleaning products we use to wipe their hands (Zahm and Ward 1998). Even manufacturing processes, like those of General Motors trucks in Flint, Michigan, emit chemicals into the air and water that hurt children. One such plant released 637,125 pounds of toxic chemicals in 2005 (Shaw 2007). A recent finding also linked childhood leukemia rates to nearby nuclear facilities (Baker and Hoel 2007). Research has shown that these exposures, among many others like vaccines, may be contributing to the rise in children's neurological developmental problems (Wakefield 2002). Autism is higher than it has ever been (Yeargin-Allsop 2003). While, like in breast cancer, there are questions of better screening and diagnosis that may make it seem like rates are going up more than is actually the case, high rates are not explained away by these factors. And autism is just one of multiple neurological misdevelopments. Others include attention deficit disorder and mental retardation (Goldman and Koduru 2000).

At the Long Island hearing, Landrigan expressed his concern not just about breast cancer but also about how the same things causing breast cancer were making children sick.

"In 1775, Sir Percivall Pott, a British surgeon, reported for the first time an association between childhood cancer and an environmental agent," he began. "Pott noted that 'climbing boys of London,' teenage boys employed as chimney sweeps, experienced a devastating incidence of cancer of the scrotum." He went on to explain how that chemicals found in the soot were the root cause of the cancer. A growing number of chemicals like benzopyrene and napthylamine were subsequently found to cause cancer in kids and adults. He referred to the recent Swedish twin study that Chafee had mentioned showing how environment was more important than genetics when it came to cancer risk.

The soot chimney sweeps once inhaled is now just one of tens of thousands of exposures in the environment today. But scientists lack basic knowledge about what their health effects are. Landrigan argued for the absolute importance of testing chemicals before they were released onto the market and the right that Americans had to know about what they were being exposed to. Regulatory standards are also not up to par. Past cases of chemical exposure like asbestos and vinyl chloride had shown that workers and communities often had no idea that toxic chemicals were entering their bodies (Markowitz and Rosner 2002).

Landrigan finished his testimony with a hard-hitting conclusion. "No longer must cancer be regarded as an inescapable consequence of aging or the result of unexplainable 'natural forces.' Quite the contrary. It is now realized that chemical carcinogenesis is not exceptional and that well over half of human cancers—perhaps as many as 80 to 90 percent worldwide—are caused by environmental exposures."

LOOK BEFORE YOU LEAP

The situation seems intractable, but it is not. There are ways to change what we are doing. Policies can be established to protect the public from these products, and new products can be developed that are safer. Two answers: the precautionary principle and green chemistry. A growing number of scientists and activists are promoting the precautionary principle, but many governments are resisting it. Jane Bright is one of those activists.

Jane was diagnosed with breast cancer when her youngest son was in high school and the older in college. She was in her early fifties. She is a composed woman with a graceful neck and upright posture. Her light brown hair is cut in a simple bangles bob, and tailored clothes hang smartly off her slim figure. "It is quite an experience to be told you have a terminal illness," Jane explained, relating her response to the diagnosis. "You start asking yourself questions that can be answered only in time, like will I see my sons graduate?" Usually when Jane speaks, she is direct and unflinching. Her hands are still, her body motionless. She has a reputation as a competent moderator and is frequently asked to lead conferences and public events. This statement, however, makes her pause, and her voice breaks as she fights tears.

For the past twenty years the Bright family has lived in Marblehead, Massachusetts, a wealthy town on the ocean north of Boston. Her sons grew up there, and Jane's career as director of human resources for a large corporation took shape then. Her husband, a quiet, mathematical man, developed a lucrative computer business during that time, and Jane eventually retired to help him develop a new product line. In the meantime, breast cancer struck, radically changing her life.

Jane had always lived a healthy lifestyle and had none of the traditional risk factors. She was mystified by the diagnosis. No one in her family had ever had breast cancer. She began to research the causes of the disease. She looked on the Web, talked to friends, and then found out about a local organization working on toxic exposures in the neighborhood.

"I had never thought about what it meant to live downwind from the power plant," said Jane. Chemicals emitted into the air from coal-burning power plants like the facility across an inlet from her house are carcinogenic (Finkelman 1999; Levy and Spengler 2000). And Marblehead has higher than state-average rates of breast cancer (as well as prostate cancer, among others). They may be related to releases from that plant. Jane had other exposures that could have caused her illness. She had endless X-rays of her upper back due to teenage scoliosis. The cosmetics she had worn, even only minimally, for many years were another concern.

As she began to understand the convoluted language and complicated aspects of parabens, PAHs, and ionizing radiation, she helped establish Health-Link, a statewide group determined to clean up the state's "filthy five" power plants. After the group helped achieve some of the most stringent air pollution regulations in the country, she was asked to join the board of the Alliance for a Healthy Tomorrow. It was launching a political and public education campaign to regulate exposures to toxic chemicals.

"Approximately 80,000 industrial chemicals are currently in commercial use in the United States. A growing body of evidence is emerging on the health impacts of exposure to some of them, but information on the effects of the vast majority of chemicals remain largely missing," states HealthLink's website. The group also maintains that "we do know that many classes of chemicals and substances, including metals, pesticides, solvents, and production byproducts, have been linked to a range of health effects, including cancer and reproductive and developmental disabilities." Many could be eliminated in a cost-effective way. Precaution and prevention are the goals.

Every year, Jane's mammogram is stultifying, frightening, and paralyzing. First, she sees her oncologist at Massachusetts General Hospital, the offices of which are high enough to look over the vast medical complex. Then she goes down two floors to the radiology unit, where the spacious external lobby is peaceful and brightly lit. The interior waiting room set apart for mammography is darker and more intimate. It is so full that several women stand. It almost seems like a salon or spa with women flipping through magazines and soft music playing in the background, except that they don't speak or look at one another. They are smothered by a worried hush and wear white medical gowns wrapped around the front.

In 2005, Jane's clean mammography meant that she had passed the five-year mark. By the American Cancer Society's standards, that makes her a survivor. But the best predictor of getting breast cancer is having had it before. Because of that, many women are more fearful of recurrence than the initial bout. Jane has coped by taking political action. This is different than the preventive actions women are offered in magazines and self-help books—those suggestions are about diet and lifestyle. Jane's life recommends transformation.

"Look before you leap" is one way to describe the philosophy that Jane espouses, otherwise called the precautionary principle. Born in Europe and spreading quickly across the United States, the precautionary principle is regarded as a defensive public health approach to reduce or ban chemicals even in the absence of understanding whether they harm human health (Krimsky 2000). Usually, the government uses risk assessment to test how many people will become ill if a chemical is released onto the market (Hertz-Picciotto 1995). Risk assessment is a type of cost-benefit analysis that uses human lives as a measurement of cost. When a manufacturer generates a new chemical and tests it for harm to human health, the analysis includes a number of human lives that will be lost. There are serious problems with this approach. First is even knowing what the risks are. A recent article in *Science* debating risk assessment posed the question, "What to do when there are no data showing, for instance, how many people became ill after exposure to a particular chemical"? (Charles 2007, 316). It is simply impossible to know how many deaths will be caused by a particular exposure, much less how many will result from the cumulative exposures from many products over a lifetime.

There are many such chemicals. While many of them have proven to be harmful, scientists still do not completely understand their health impacts. Massachusetts activists have worked hard to pass a bill in the state legislature to prevent pesticide spraying. In 2002, California activists pushed for the passage of a precautionary principle ordinance for the city of San Francisco (Breast Cancer Fund 2003). It mandates that governmental expenditures be directed toward more sustainable products. For example, the purchase of chlorine-based products is disallowed. A group of organizations on Long Island created a similar campaign. State or local governments have taken some action. The European Union has taken more.

The European Union was one of the first governments to begin to implement the precautionary principle (Gremmen and van den Belt 2000) and has banned phthalates and other chemicals (Vogel 2000). In 2002, it implemented an ordinance barring manufacturers from selling cosmetics that used those or a number of other carcinogenic ingredients. The European Union gave companies two years to replace the chemicals with something safer. Aveda, Urban Decay, Neways International, and The Body Shop had voluntarily followed suit in the United States. Osea Skin Care and Avalon Natural Products were already making products without the newly banned ingredients.

American cosmetics companies have faced challenges from women in their own country who do not want these chemicals in makeup. But the U.S. government has taken little action to exclude them from production. For example, the Food and Drug Administration does little to regulate those contents. With the passage of the new EU policy, manufacturers had to decide if they would continue to produce the same cosmetics for the American market while making safer chemicals for the European Union or to completely phase out phthalates and other similar ingredients. Most large cosmetics manufacturers—Avon, Revlon, and Maybelline—decided to take the first approach (Malkan 2008). Recently, a smattering of these companies announced that they would remove phthalates from their products, but there are many more potentially hazardous ingredients to go.

Decreasing exposure to these chemicals could mean lowering cancer rates. But if we stop using these chemicals, what will we use instead?

GREEN CHEMISTRY

Looking before you leap has massive ramifications. In some instances, it may mean that there is no product or drug available or affordable when needed. These are some of the reasons why it is difficult for the precautionary principle to be put into action. The precautionary principle does not provide a set of alternatives but rather reduces risk. Putting the precautionary principle in place must be supplemented by new production practices that work better. That is where green chemistry comes in. Green chemistry is a set of concepts and principles underlying the production of chemicals that was developed in the 1990s when Joe Breen founded the U.S. Green Chemistry Institute. Aimed at reducing hazardous waste, it has produced alternative chemical processes and products that do not harm human health, such as new catalysts, safer chemicals and environmentally benign solvents, and renewable feedstocks (Anastas and Kirchhoff 2002).

One of the principles of green chemistry is to reduce the waste and hazards created in the production process. Generally, new "catalysts" are developed that radically change the impact of industrial production. Catalysts are chemicals or processes used during the creation of a product. It is not only products themselves that need to be fixed but also the pollutants emitted during their production. For example, Pfizer, one of the largest pharmaceutical companies in the world, developed a new catalytic process for making the active ingredient sertraline in its popular antidepressant Zoloft (Ritter 2002). Scientists at the famous and widely celebrated Los Alamos plant in New Mexico are working on such projects, several of them that massively reduce energy usage. Other scientists there are collaborating with companies to develop fuel cells for phones that run on methanol. These are just a few of many changes. Green chemistry has expanded globally in the past fifteen years. National governments, industry, and academic researchers are all innovating with its techniques (Tundo et al. 2000).

Breen was pictured in a 2002 *Science* article that commemorated his work (Poliakoff et al. 2002). Tall and thin, his wiry beard falls across a black suit cleaned with a novel carbon dioxide process rather than dry cleaning, which uses perchloroethylene, a highly toxic ingredient. Called "DryClean" in the industry, his carbon dioxide product is powerful and less toxic. This product is used in other production processes as well, like removing caffeine from coffee, rather than using noxious chemicals like formaldehyde. This "supercritical" carbon dioxide is also an improvement on other chemicals used as catalysts in production processes, resulting in improved energy efficiency.

Born in the 1940s in Connecticut, Breen grew up during the period that chemicals began to proliferate around the planet. As much as anyone, he was faced with these chemicals during the twenty years he worked at the U.S. Environmental Protection Agency. It was not until he retired that he had the time to found the green chemistry movement, which almost immediately blossomed in unexpected ways. The excitement and controversy over green chemistry has spread from lab to boardroom to newspaper headline. Breast cancer activists concerned about chemical exposures are on board. The Breast Cancer Fund (2006) has argued that "all constituents who care about the future of the state must come together to develop a unified plan to manage hazardous chemicals in our environment" and that green chemistry is critical to that plan.

THE FUTURE OF BREAST CANCER'S SCIENTIFIC ECONOMY

Julia Brody, Jane Houlihan, Theo Colburn, Zena Werb, and a long list of others have shifted the science of breast cancer. Most researchers have been hemmed in by the scientific economy of the disease, funded to research about cure and treatment, and using the tools standard to biomedical research. But they have moved in new directions, constructing new tools, testing new hypotheses, and discovering new toxics. Their research has received harsh criticism, and their professional credibility has been challenged. Women with breast cancer have both supported them and asked for more. Surrounded by incessant illness and death, these women know only too well that time is of the essence.

Women who have become activists often realize that science is slow. In contacting corporate representatives who refuse to return their calls or answer their concerns, they cannot help but understand the entrenched nature of the political economy of disease. Political economy is also interrelated with the minutiae of science. And so activists have served on review panels and advised scientists about environmental links to breast cancer, trying to shift that too. They have educated, persuaded, demonstrated, and, above all, persisted. They have not taken no for an answer, nor should we.

The critiques offered in this book are not meant to make anyone look bad. Rather, they are directed toward changing the machines of production causing ill health in America. No one individual or even one company has created this situation. Nor can any one radically alter it. Americans must form a rising tide where individuals ask for safer products, demand to know ingredients, and educate themselves about where their hard-earned dollars go. This sea change is already taking place, although it is dwarfed by massive industries that have yet to take note. There are dollars and lives on the line. To the everyday Jane, life is of the utmost importance. To the everyday Dollar Bill Corporation, it is profits. These two agendas can be brought into line with one another. It is simply a matter of demanding it.

Every eleven minutes, an American woman dies of breast cancer. We can change that.

Robin had finished reconstructive surgery and recovered. We had stopped shooting for the film months ago. I had not spoken to her and lost track of what the family was planning and how she was feeling. Summer was just beginning as spring blooms fell away under dazzling sunlight. It was almost three years since I had met Robin. That was a long time to follow someone around, peering into her life. She had shared a lot with me, and we had actually gotten to be friends.

I decided to call. Her voice mail confronted me. She didn't call back. Usually I heard from her within a day or two at the most. I called again. This time she responded by e-mail.

"So sorry, Brina. Things are bad. I found another lump. I'll have it out this week. Deciding between aggressive chemo and radiation. So many opinions. I don't know." My stomach heaved. Watching her go through months of chemotherapy was painful. I could not imagine how she could face it again. "I'll be okay, I know. XO, Robin," her e-mail finished. She still had such an optimistic outlook. She refused to be beaten—one obstacle after another, this one possibly the toughest.

Appendix: Resource List

Alliance For a Healthy Tomorrow c/o Clean Water Action
262 Washington Street
Room 301
Boston, MA 02108
tel.: 617-338-8131
www.healthytomorrow.org

Breast Cancer Action
55 New Montgomery Street
Suite 323
San Francisco, CA 94105
tel.: 877-2STOPBC (877-278-6722)
www.bcaction.org

Breast Cancer Fund
1388 Sutter Street
Suite 400
San Francisco, CA 94109-5400
tel.: 415-346-8223, 866-760-8223
www.breastcancerfund.org

Clean Water Action
262 Washington
Suite 301

Boston, MA 02108
tel.: 617-654-8284
fax: 617-338-6449
www.cleanwateraction.org

The Collaborative on Health and Environment
c/o Commonweal
PO Box 316
Bolinas, CA 94924
www.healthandenvironment.org

The Environmental Working Group
Headquarters
1436 U Street NW
Suite 100
Washington, DC 20009
tel.: 202-667-6982
California Office
2201 Broadway
Suite 308
Oakland, CA 94612
tel.: 510-444-0973
www.ewg.org

HealthLink
60 Monument Avenue
PO Box 301
Swampscott, MA 01907
tel.: 781-598-1115
www.HealthLink.org

Huntington Breast Cancer Action Coalition
746 New York Avenue
Huntington, NY 11743
tel.: 631-547-1518
fax: 631-547-1520
www.hbcac.org

Massachusetts Breast Cancer Coalition
1419 Hancock Street
Suite 202

Quincy, MA 02169
tel.: 617-376-6222
fax: 617-376-6221
www.mbcc.org

Prevention Is the Cure
746 New York Avenue
PO Box 1446
Huntington, NY 11743
tel.: 631-547-1518
fax: 631-547-1520
www.preventionisthecure.org

Silent Spring Institute
29 Crafts Street
Newton, MA 02458
tel.: 617-332-4288
fax: 617-332-4284
www.silentspring.org

Women's Health and Environment Network
704 North 23rd Street
Philadelphia, PA 19130
tel.: 215-990-1271
www.when.org

References

Aisenberg, Alan C., Dianne M. Finkelstein, Karen P. Doppke, Frederick C. Koerner, Jean-François Boivin, and Christopher G. Willett. 1997. High risk of breast carcinoma after irradiation of young women with Hodgkin's disease. *Cancer* 79, no. 6: 1203–10.

Albrektsen, G., I. Heuch, and G. Kvale. 1995. The short-term and long-term effect of a pregnancy on breast cancer risk: A prospective study of 802,457 parous Norwegian women. *British Journal of Cancer* 72: 480–84.

Altman, R. 1996. *Waking up, fighting back: The politics of breast cancer*. Boston: Little, Brown.

Ambrosone, C. B. 2001. Impact of genetics on the relationship between smoking and breast cancer risk. *Journal of Women's Cancer* 3: 17–22.

American Cancer Society. 2005. National Home Office Form 990. Tax document. Atlanta: American Cancer Society.

———. 2006a. Detailed guide: Male breast cancer. What are the key statistics about breast cancer in men? Atlanta: American Cancer Society.

———. 2006b. *Lifestyle vs. breast cancer: The role of food, fitness, and weight in your risk of breast cancer*. http://www.cancer.org/docroot/NWS/content/NWS_1_1x _Lifestyle_vs_Breast_Cancer.asp

———. 2007. *Cancer Facts and Figures 2007*. Atlanta: American Cancer Society.

———. 2008. *Cancer Facts and Figures 2008*. Atlanta: American Cancer Society.

Anastas, Paul T., and Mary M. Kirchhoff. 2002. Origins, current status, and future challenges of green chemistry. *Accounts of Chemical Research* 35, no. 9: 686–94.

Anderson, David E. 1976. *Risk factors in breast cancer*. Chicago: Year Book Medical Publishers.

Angell, Marcia. 2004. *The truth about the drug companies: How they deceive us and what to do about it*. New York: Random House.

Angier, Natalie. 1994. Fierce competition marked fervid race for cancer gene. *New York Times*, Sept. 20.

Anglin, Mary K. 1997. Working from the inside out: Implications of breast cancer activism for biomedical policies and practices. *Social Science and Medicine* 44: 1403–15.

Ardies, C., and C. Dees. 1998. Xenoestrogens significantly enhance risk for breast cancer during growth and adolescence. *Medical Hypotheses* 50, no. 6: 457–64.

Arlidge, John. 1999. Polluters named and shamed: Healthcare giants among factories emitting 400,000 tonnes of toxic waste a year. *The Observer* (London), May 30.

Arnold, S. F., P. M. Vonier, B. M. Collins, D. M. Klotz, L. J. Guillette Jr., and J. A. McLachlan. 1997. *In vitro* synergistic interaction of alligator and human estrogen receptors with combinations of environmental chemicals. *Environmental Health Perspectives* 105, suppl. 3: 615–18.

Aronson, Kristan J., Anthony B. Miller, Christy G. Woolcott, Ernest E. Sterns, David R. McCready, Lavina A. Lickley, Edward B. Fish, George Y. Hiraki, Claire Holloway, Ted Ross, Wedad M. Hanna, Sandip K. SenGupta, and Jean-Phillipe Weber. 2000. Breast adipose tissue concentrations of polychlorinated biphenyls and other organochlorines and breast cancer risk. *Cancer Epidemiology, Biomarkers and Prevention* 9: 55–63.

Aschengrau, A., P. F. Coogan, M. Quinn, and L. J. Cashins. 1998. Occupational exposure to estrogenic chemicals and the occurrence of breast cancer: An exploratory analysis. *American Journal of Industrial Medicine* 34: 6–14.

Aschengrau, A., and D. Ozonoff. 1992. *Upper Cape Cod Cancer Incidence Study: Final report*. Boston: Massachusetts Department of Public Health.

AstraZeneca. 2004. *Annual review*. London: AstraZeneca.

——. 2006. *Annual review and highlight of financial statements*. London: AstraZeneca.

Avon Corporation. 2003. *Annual report*. New York: Avon Corporation.

Baker, P. J., and D. Hoel. 2007. Meta-analysis of standardized incidence and mortality rates of childhood leukaemia in proximity to nuclear facilities. *European Journal of Cancer Care* 16: 355–63.

Barbone, Fabio, Rosa Filiberti, Silvia Franceschi, Renato Talamini, Ettore Conti, Maurizio Montella, and Carlo La Vecchia. 1996. Socioeconomic status, migration and the risk of breast cancer in Italy. *International Journal of Epidemiology* 25, no. 3: 479–87.

Batt, Sharon. 1995. *Patient no more: The politics of breast cancer*. Charlottetown, PE: Gynergy Books.

Batt, Sharon, and Liza Gross. 1999. Cancer, Inc. *Sierra Magazine*, September/October. http://www.sierraclub.org/sierra/199909/cancer.asp

BBC News. 1998. *US backs Tamoxifen as cancer prevention treatment*. http://news .bbc.co.uk/2/hi/health/163577.stm

Berkeley City Council. 2003. *Precautionary principle ordinance (CF 36-04)*. http:// www.ci.berkeley.ca.us/citycouncil/2005citycouncil/packet/051005/2005-05 -10%20Item%2025.pdf

Bernard, Alfred, Sylviane Carbonnelle, Claire de Burbure, Olivier Michel, and Marc Nickmilder. 2006. Chlorinated pool attendance, atopy, and the risk of asthma during childhood. *Environmental Health Perspectives* 114: 1567–73.

Birnbaum, Linda S., and Suzanne E. Fenton. 2003. Cancer and developmental exposure to endocrine disruptors. *Environmental Health Perspectives* 111: 389–94.

Blackledge, George. 2002. AstraZeneca's Hormone Portfolio. PowerPoint presentation.

Boice, J. D., Jr. 2001. Radiation and breast carcinogenesis. *Medical and Pediatric Oncology* 36: 508–13.

Boice, J. D., Jr., C. E. Land, and D. L. Preston. 1996. Ionizing radiation. In *Cancer epidemiology and prevention*, edited by D. Schottenfeld and J. F. Fraumeni Jr. New York: Oxford University Press, 319–54.

Bonadonna, Gianni, Pinuccia Valagussa, Angela Moliterni, Milvia Zambetti, and Cristina Brambilla. 1995. Adjuvant cyclophosphamide, methotrexate, and fluorouracil in node-positive breast cancer—The results of 20 years of follow-up. *New England Journal of Medicine* 332: 901–6.

Boseley, Sarah. 2006. Drug firms a danger to health—Report: International research exposes flaws in £33bn marketing budget. *The Guardian*, June 26.

Bradbury, A., and O. Olopade. 2006. The case for individualized screening recommendations for breast cancer. *Journal of Clinical Oncology* 24, no. 21: 3328.

Braun, Lundy. 2003. Engaging the experts: Popular science education and breast cancer activism. *Critical Public Health* 13, no. 3: 191–206.

Breast Cancer Action. 2003. http://www.thinkbeforeyoupink.org/Pages/PrettyInPink.html (accessed February 12, 2004).

Breast Cancer and Environmental Risk Factors. 2004. BCERF EnviroChem and Cancer Database. *The Ribbon Newsletter* 9, no. 3: 1.

Breast Cancer Fund. 2000. Breast cancer: Is it the environment? *MS Magazine*, April/May.

Brenner, Barbara. 2000. Sister Support: Women create a breast cancer movement. In *Breast cancer: Society shapes an epidemic*, edited by A. S. Kasper and S. J. Ferguson. New York: Palgrave, 325–54.

———. 2002. From the executive director: The Wild, Wild West of women's health. *Breast Cancer Action Newsletter*, no. 73 (September/October), http://bcaction.org/index.php?page=newsletter-73c

Brodie, M. 2001. *Understanding the effects of direct-to-consumer prescription drug advertising*. Menlo Park, CA: Henry J. Kaiser Family Foundation.

Brody, J. G., and R. A. Rudel. 2003. Environmental pollutants and breast cancer. *Environmental Health Perspectives* 111: 1007–19.

Brody, J. G., D. J. Vorhees, S. J. Melly, S. R. Swedis, P. J. Drivas, and R. A. Rudel. 2002. Using GIS and historical records to reconstruct residential exposure to large-scale pesticide application. *Journal of Exposure Analysis and Environmental Epidemiology* 12: 64–80.

Brown, Phil, and Judith Kirwan Kelley. 2000. Physicians' knowledge, attitudes and practice regarding environmental health hazards. In *Illness and the environment: A reader in contested medicine*, edited by J. Stephen Kroll-Smith, Phil Brown, and Valerie Jan Gunter. New York: New York University Press.

Brown, Phil, Sabrina McCormick, Brian Mayer, Stephen Zavestoski, Rachel Morello-Frosch, Rebecca Gasior Altman, and Laura Senier. 2006. "A lab of our own": Environmental causation of breast cancer and challenges to the dominant epidemiological paradigm. *Science, Technology, and Human Values* 31, no. 5: 499–536.

Brown, Phil, and Edwin Mikkelsen. 1990. *No Safe Place: Toxic waste, leukemia, and community action.* Berkeley: University of California Press.

Brown, Phil, Stephen Zavestoski, Sabrina McCormick, Joshua Mandelbaum, and Theo Luebke. 2001. Print media coverage of environmental causation of breast cancer. *Sociology of Health and Illness* 23, no. 6: 747–75.

Buell, P. 1973. Changing incidence of breast cancer in Japanese-American women. *Journal of the National Cancer Institute* 51: 1479–83.

Busfield, Joan. 2007. Pills, power, people: Sociological understandings of the pharmaceutical industry. In *Perspectives in medical sociology*, 4th ed., edited by Phil Brown. Long Grove, IL: Waveland Press.

Bu-Tian Ji, Aaron Blair, Xiao-Ou Shu, Wong-Ho Chow, Michael Hauptmann, Mustafa Dosemeci, Gong Yang, Jay Lubin, Yu-Tang Gao, Nathaniel Rothma, and Wei Zheng. 2008. Occupation and breast cancer risk among Shanghai women in a population-based cohort study. *American Journal of Industrial Medicine* 51: 100–110.

Canadian Institutes of Health Research. 2002. *Identifying national research priorities for the environmental influences on health.* http://www.cihr-irsc.gc.ca/e/pdf_14818.htm

Caplan, L. S., E. R. Schoenfeld, E. S. O'Leary, and M. C. Leske. 2000. Breast cancer and electromagnetic fields—A review. *Annals of Epidemiology* 10, no. 1: 31–44.

Caporaso, James A., and David P. Levine. 1992. *Theories of political economy.* Cambridge: Cambridge University Press.

Carson, Rachel. 1961. *Silent spring.* New York: Houghton Mifflin.

Casamayou, Maureen Hogan. 2001. *The politics of breast cancer.* Washington, DC: Georgetown University Press.

Castells, Manuel. 1997. *The power of identity.* Malden, MA: Blackwell.

Cause Marketing Forum. 2003. *2003 Cause Marketing Halo Award winners.* http://www.causemarketingforum.com/page.asp?ID=77

———. 2007. *The growth of cause marketing.* http://www.causemarketingforum.com/page.asp?ID=188

Caywood, Thomas. 2004. Tests find toxins in Cape homes' air. *Boston Herald*, November 18.

Center for Policy Alternatives. 2000. *Playing fair: State action to lower prescription drug prices.* Washington, DC: Center for Policy Alternatives.

Centers for Disease Control and Prevention. 2003. *Second national report on human exposures to carcinogens.* Atlanta: Centers for Disease Control and Prevention. http://www.cdc.gov/exposurereport

Charles, Daniel. 2007. Regulatory science: Panel pans proposed change in U.S. risk assessment. *Science* 19, no. 5810: 316.

Cirlot, J. E. 1971. *A dictionary of symbols*, translated by Jack Sage. New York: Philosophical Library. (Spanish ed. 1962).

Clark, Claudia. 1997. *Radium girls: Women and industrial health reform, 1910–1935.* Chapel Hill: University of North Carolina Press.

Clark, Rachel Ann, Suzanne Snedeker, and Carol Devine. 1998. *Estrogen and breast cancer risk: The relationship: Fact sheet #09. Breast cancer and environment risk factors*. Ithaca, NY: Cornell University.

Clarke, Christina A., Sally L. Glaser, Dee W. West, Rochelle R. Ereman, Christine A. Erdmann, Janice M. Barlow, and Margaret R. Wrensch. 2002. Breast cancer incidence and mortality trends in an affluent population: Marin County, California, USA, 1990–1999. *Breast Cancer Research* 4, no. 6: R13.

Clorfene-Casten, Liane. 1996. *Breast cancer, poisons, profits and prevention*. Monroe, ME: Common Courage Press.

Colborn, Theo, Dianne Dumanoski, and John P. Myers. 2002. *Our stolen future: Are we threatening our fertility, intelligence, and survival?* New York: Penguin Books.

Colborn, T., F. S. vom Saal, and Anna M. Soto. 1993. Developmental effects of endocrine disrupting chemicals in wildlife and humans. *Environmental Health Perspectives* 101: 378–84.

Colditz, G. A., and B. Rosner. (2000). Cumulative risk of breast cancer to age 70 years according to risk factor status: Data from the Nurses' Health Study. *American Journal of Epidemiology* 152: 950.

Collaborative Group on Hormonal Factors in Breast Cancer. 2002. Breast cancer and breastfeeding: Collaborative reanalysis of individual data from 47 epidemiological studies in 30 countries, including 50,302 women with breast cancer and 96,973 women without the disease. *Lancet* 360: 187–95.

Commission of European Communities. 2004. *The European Environment and Health Action Plan 2004–2010*. Brussels: Commission of European Communities.

Committee on Science. 2002. *Environmental contributors to breast cancer: What does the science say?* Field Hearing before the Subcommittee on Environment, Technology and Standards Committee on Science, House of Representatives. http://commdocs.house.gov/committees/science/hsy80226.000/hsy80226_0.htm

Congressionally Directed Medical Research Programs. 2003. *Breast cancer*. Department of Defense. http://cdmrp.army.mil/bcrp.

Conrad, Peter. 1999. A mirage of genes. *Sociology of Health and Illness* 21, no 2: 228–41.

Correa, Adolfo, Ronald H. Gray, Rebecca Cohen, Nathaniel Rothman, Faridah Shah, Hui Seacat and Morton Com. 1996. Ethylene glycol ethers and risks of spontaneous abortion and subfertility. *American Journal of Epidemiology* 143: 707–17.

Damstra, T., S. Barlow, A. Bergman, R. Kavlock, and G. Van Der Kraak, eds. 2002. Global assessment of the state-of-the-science of endocrine disruptors. International Programme on Chemical Safety. http://ehp.niehs.nih.gov/who

Daniel, Pete. 2006. Toxic drift: The lasting legacy of post-World War II pesticide use. Division of Work and Industry, Smithsonian National Museum of American History.

Davis, Devra. 2002. *When smoke ran like water: Tales of environmental deception and the battle against pollution*. New York: Basic Books.

Davis, Devra Lee, and H. Leon Bradlow. 1995. Can environmental estrogens cause breast cancer? *Scientific American*, Fall, 144–49.

Davis, Devra L., H. Leon Bradlow, Mary Wolff, T. Woodruff, D. G. Hoel, and H. Anton-Culver. 1993. Medical hypothesis: Xenoestrogens as preventable causes of breast cancer. *Environmental Health Perspectives* 101: 372–77.

Davis, Devra, and Pamela Webster. 2002. The social context of science: Cancer and the environment. *Annals of the American Academy of Political and Social Science* 584: 13–34.

Deapen, Dennis, Lihua Liu, Carin Perkins, Leslie Bernstein, and Ronald K. Ross. 2002. Rapidly rising breast cancer incidence rates among Asian-American women. *International Journal of Cancer* 99, no. 5: 747–50.

DeBruin, L. S., and P. D. Josephy. 2002. Perspectives on the chemical etiology of breast cancer. *Environmental Health Perspectives* 110, suppl. 1: 119–28.

Department of Health and Human Services. 2007. *Policy issues associated with undertaking a new large U.S. population cohort study of genes, environment, and disease.* Washington, DC: Secretary's Advisory Committee on Genetics, Health, and Society.

Destounis, Stamatia V., Patricia DiNitto, Wende Logan-Young, Ermelinda Bonaccio, Margarita L. Zuley, and Kathleen M. Willison. 2004. Can computer-aided detection with double reading of screening mammograms help decrease the false-negative rate? Initial experience. *Radiology* 232: 578–84.

Dewailly, Éric, Sylvie Dodin, René Verreault, Pierre Ayotte, Louise Sauvé, Jacques Morin, and Jacques Brisson. 1994. High organochlorine body burden in women with estrogen receptor-positive breast cancer. *Journal of the National Cancer Institute* 86: 232–34.

DiMaggio, Paul J., and Walter W. Powell. 1983. The iron cage revisited: Institutional isomorphism and collective rationality in organizational fields. *American Sociological Review* 48: 147–60.

Doody, Michele Morin, John E. Lonstein, Marilyn Stovall, David G. Hacker, Nickolas Luckyanov, and Charles E. Land. 2000. Breast cancer mortality after diagnostic radiography: Findings from the U.S. Scoliosis Cohort Study. *Spine* 25, no. 16: 2052–63.

Dorgan, J., John Brock, Nathaniel Rothman, Larry Needham, Rosetta Miller, Hugh E. Stephenson, Nicki Schussler, and Philip R. Taylor. 1999. Serum organochlorine pesticides and PCBs and breast cancer risk: Results from a prospective analysis. *Cancer Causes and Control* 10: 1–11.

Dow Jones Business Wire. Iron mountain mine superfund site settlement. 2000.

Dunnick, Reed. 2005. Better quality for women in screening sites. *Saving women's lives: Strategies for improving breast cancer detection and diagnosis—A Breast Cancer Research Foundation and Institute of Medicine Symposium.* Washington, DC: National Cancer Policy Board.

Ehrenreich, Barbara. 2001. Welcome to cancerland: A mammogram leads to a cult of pink kitsch. *Harper's Magazine*, November, 43–53.

Eisen, Andrea, and Barbara L. Weber. 1999. Prophylactic mastectomy—The price of fear. *New England Journal of Medicine* 340: 137–38.

Environmental Protection Agency. 2000. *EPA's health assessment.* Washington, DC: Environmental Protection Agency.

Environmental Working Group. 2003. *Bodyburden: The pollution in people*. Washington, DC: Environmental Working Group.

——. 2008. *Skin deep database: Avon Breast Cancer Crusade Limited-Edition Celebrity Crusade Nailwear Nail Enamel*. http://www.cosmeticsdatabase.com/product.php?prod_id=60171

Epstein, Samuel S., Barbara Seaman, and Rosalie Bertell. 2001. Dangers and unreliability of mammography: Breast examination is a safe, effective and practical alternative. *International Journal of Health Services* 31, no. 3: 605–15.

Estée Lauder Companies. 2005. *Annual report*. New York: Estée Lauder, Inc.

Evans, Nancy, ed. 2006. *The state of the evidence: What is the connection between breast cancer and the environment?* San Francisco: The Breast Cancer Fund.

Fagin, Dan. 2002. Tattered hopes. Three-part series. *Newsday*, July 28–30.

Fagin, Dan, and Marianne Lavelle. 1996. *Toxic deception: How the chemical industry manipulates science, bends the law and endangers your health*. Secaucus, NJ: Carol Publishing Group.

Fernandez, Sandy M. 1998. Pretty in pink—The history of the pink ribbon. *MAMM*, June/July.

File, Karen Maru, and Russ Alan Prince. 2004. Cause related marketing and corporate philanthropy in the privately held enterprise. *Journal of Business Ethics* 17, no. 14: 1529–1539.

Fine, P. 2004. Review of *Cholera, chloroform and the science of medicine: A life of John Snow*, by Peter Vinten-Johansen, Howard Brody, Nigel Paneth, Stephen Rachkman, and Michael Rip (with David Zuck). *Public Health* 118, no. 6: 453–53.

Finkelman, Robert B. 1999. Trace elements in coal: Environmental and health significance. *Biological Trace Element Research* 67, no. 3: 197–204.

Fisher, Bernard. 1970. The surgical dilemma in the primary therapy of invasive breast cancer: A critical appraisal. *Current Problems in Surgery*, 3–53.

——. 1997. Highlights of the NSABP Breast Cancer Prevention Trial. *Cancer Control* 4, no. 1: 78–86.

Food and Drug Administration. 1995. *FDA authority over cosmetics*. Center for Food Safety and Applied Nutrition. Office of Cosmetics and Colors. http://www.cfsan.fda.gov/~dms/cos-206.html

Ford, Leslie. 1998. *Testimony on the Breast Cancer Prevention Trial*. Congressional Caucus for Women's Issues. http://legislative.cancer.gov/files/testimony-1998-04-30.pdf

Gammon, M. D., R. M. Santella, A. I. Neugut, S. M. Eng, S. L. Teitelbaum, A. Paykin, B. Levin, M. B. Terry, T. L. Young, L. W. Wang, Q. Wang, J. A. Britton, M. S. Wolff, S. D. Stellman, M. Hatch, G. C. Kabat, R. Senie, G. Garbowksi, C. Maffeo, P. Montalvan, G. Berkowitz, M. Kemeny, M. Citron, F. Schnabel, A. Schuss, S. Hajdu, and V. Vinceguerra. 2002a. Environmental toxins and breast cancer on Long Island. Polycyclic aromatic hydrocarbon DNA adducts. *Cancer Epidemiology Biomarkers and Prevention* 11: 677–85.

Gammon, M. D., M. S. Wolff, A. I. Neugut, S. M. Eng, S. L. Teitelbaum, J. A. Britton, M. B. Terry, B. Levin, S. D. Stellman, G. C. Kabat, M. Hatch, R. Senie, G. Berkowitz, H. L. Bradlow, G. Garbowski, C. Maffeo, P. Montalvan, M. Kemeny, M. Citron, F. Schnabel, A. Schuss, S. Hajdu, V. Vinceguerra, N. Niguidula, K. Ireland,

and R. M. Santella. 2002b. Environmental toxins and breast cancer on Long Island. II. Organochlorine compound levels in blood. *Cancer Epidemiology, Biomarkers and Prevention* 11: 686–97.

Gardner, Kirsten E. 2006. *Early detection: Women, cancer, and awareness campaigns in the twentieth-century United States*. Chapel Hill: University of North Carolina Press.

Givel, Michael, and Stanton A. Glantz. 2004. The "global settlement" with the tobacco industry: 6 years later. *American Journal of Public Health* 94, no. 2: 218–24.

Gledhill, Linda. 2005. Migden's cosmetics bill OK'd by health committee: Chemicals would be catalogued online. *SF Chronicle*, sec. B, June 29.

Goldberg, M. S., and F. Labrèche. (1996). Occupational risk factors for female breast cancer: A review. *Occupational and Environmental Medicine* 53: 145–56.

Goldhirsch, Aron, John H. Glick, Richard D. Gelber, Alan S. Coates, and Hans-Jörg Senn. 2001. Meeting highlights: International Consensus Panel on the Treatment of Primary Breast Cancer. *Journal of Clinical Oncology* 19, no. 18: 3817–27.

Goldman, Lynn R., and S. Koduru. 2000. Chemicals in the environment and developmental toxicity to children: A public health and policy perspective. *Environmental Health Perspectives* 108, suppl. 3: 443–48.

Graphic Artists Guild. 2006. *Pricing and ethical guidelines*. 11th ed. New York: Northlight Books.

Greenwald, P. 1999. Role of dietary fat in the causation of breast cancer: Point. *Cancer Epidemiology, Biomarkers and Prevention* 8: 3–7.

Gremmen, Bart, and Henk van den Belt. 2000. The precautionary principle and pesticides. *Journal of Agricultural and Environmental Ethics* 12, no. 2: 197–205.

Guillette, L. J., Jr., T. S. Gross, G. R. Masson, J. M. Matter, J. M., H. F. Percival, and A. R. Woodward. 1994. Developmental abnormalities of the gonad and abnormal sex hormone concentrations in juvenile alligators from contaminated and control lakes in Florida. *Environmental Health Perspectives* 102: 680–88.

Guttes, K. Failing, K. Neumann, J. Kleinstein, S. Georgii, and H. Brunn. 1998. Chlororganic pesticides and polychlorinated biphenyls in breast tissue of women with benign and malignant breast disease. *Archives of Environmental Contamination and Toxicology* 35, no. 1: 140–47.

Hackshaw, A. K., and E. A. Paul. 2003. Breast self-examination and death from breast cancer: A meta-analysis. *British Journal of Cancer* 88: 1047–53.

Hadjiiski, Lubomir, Heang-Ping Chan, Berkman Sahiner, Mark A. Helvie, Marilyn A. Roubidoux, Caroline Blane, Chintana Paramagul, Nicholas Petrick, Janet Bailey, Katherine Klein, Michelle Foster, Stephanie Patterson, Dorit Adler, Alexis Nees, and Joseph Shen. 2004. Improvement in radiologists' characterization of malignant and benign breast masses on serial mammograms with computer-aided diagnosis: An ROC study. *Radiology* 233: 255–65.

Hankinson, Susan E., W. C. Willett, G. A. Colditz, D. J. Hunter, D. S. Michaud, B. Denoo, B. Rosner, F. E. Speizer, and M. Pollak. 1998. Circulating concentrations of insulin-like growth factor-I and risk of breast cancer. *Lancet* 351: 1393–96.

Hansen, Johnni. 1999. Breast cancer risk among relatively young women employed in solvent-using industries. *American Journal of Industrial Medicine* 36: 43–47.

Harvey, Philip W., and Philippa Darbre. 2004. Endocrine disrupters and human health: Could oestrogenic chemicals in body care cosmetics adversely affect breast cancer incidence in women? *Journal of Applied Toxicology* 24, no. 3: 167–76.

Hensel, Bill, Jr. 2002. Pollution lawsuit a drain on port; Director cites legal fees in reduction of net income. *Houston Chronicle*.

Hertz-Picciotto, I. 1995. Epidemiology and quantitative risk assessment: A bridge from science to policy. *American Journal of Public Health* 85, no. 4: 484–91.

Houlihan, Jane, Charlotte Brody, and Bryony Schwan. 2002. *Not too pretty: Phthalates, beauty products and the FDA.* Washington, DC: Environmental Working Group.

House of Representatives. 1993. http://www.house.gov/lantos/html_files/womens _protecting.html

Høyer, A. P., T. Jørgensen, J. W. Brock, and P. Grandjean. 2000. Organochlorine exposure and breast cancer survival. *Journal of Clinical Epidemiology* 53, no. 3: 323–30.

Hunter, David J., Susan Hankinson, Francine Laden, Graham Colditz, JoAnn E. Manson, Walter Willett, Frank Speizer, and Mary S. Wolff. 1997. Plasma organochlorine levels and the risk of breast cancer. *New England Journal of Medicine* 337: 1253–58.

Institute of Medicine. 2001. *Mammography and beyond: Developing technologies for the early detection of breast cancer.* Washington, DC: National Academies Press.

Ismail, M. Asif. 2005. *Drug lobby second to none: How the pharmaceutical industry gets its way in Washington.* Washington, DC: Center for Public Integrity.

Jenkins, Sarah, Craig Rowell, Jun Wang, and Coral A. Lamartiniere. 1999. Prenatal TCDD exposure predisposes for mammary cancer in rats. *Reproductive Toxicology* 23, no. 3: 391–96.

Johnson-Thompson, Marian C., and Janet Guthrie. 2000. Ongoing research to identify environmental risk factors in breast carcinoma. *Cancer* 88, suppl. 5: 1224–29.

Kajekar, Radhika. 2007. Environmental factors and developmental outcomes in the lung. *Pharmacology and Therapeutics* 114, no. 2: 129–45.

Kelsey, J. L., and L. Bernstein. 1996. Epidemiology and prevention of breast cancer. *Annual Review of Public Health* 17: 47–67.

Kerlikowske, K., D. Grady, J. Barclay, E. A. Sickles, and V. Ernster. 1996. Effect of age, breast density, and family history on the sensitivity of first screening mammography. *Journal of the American Medical Association* 2761: 33–38.

Khalili N. R., P. A. Scheff, and T. M. Holsen. 1995. PAH source fingerprints for coke ovens, diesel and gasoline engines, highway tunnels, and wood combustion emissions. *Atmospheric Environment* 29, no. 4: 533–42.

King, Mary-Claire, Joan H. Marks, and Jessica B. Mandell. 2003. Breast and ovarian cancer risks due to inherited mutations in *BRCA1* and *BRCA2*. *Science* 302, no. 5645: 643–46.

King, S. 2006. *Pink Ribbons, Inc.: Breast cancer and the politics of philanthropy.* Minneapolis: University of Minnesota Press.

Knorr-Cetina, K. 1999. *Epistemic cultures: How the sciences make knowledge.* Cambridge, MA: Harvard University Press.

Kolata, Gina. 1988. Smoking and cancer: What cigarette concerns really knew. *New York Times*, June 17. http://query.nytimes.com/gst/fullpage.html?sec=health&res =940DE0DA153DF934A25755C0A96E948260

———. 1997. DDT and breast cancer. *New York Times*. November 2.

———. 2002. The Epidemic that Wasn't. *The New York Times*, August 29.

Kolker, Emily S. 2004. Framing as a cultural resource in health social movements: Funding activism and the breast cancer movement in the U.S. 1990–1993. *Sociology of Health and Illness* 26, no. 6: 820–44.

Komen for the Cure. 2006. *2006 Form 990 Parent Return*. Dallas: Komen Foundation.

———. 2007a. http://cms.komen.org/komen/AboutUs/SusanGKomensStory/index .htm

———. 2007b. *Annual report*. Dallas: Susan G. Komen for the Cure.

Kopans, Daniel B. 1992. The positive predictive value of mammography. *American Journal of Roentgenology* 153: 521–26.

Krimsky, Sheldon. 2000. *Hormonal chaos: The scientific and social origins of the environmental endocrine hypothesis*. Baltimore: Johns Hopkins University Press.

———. 2003. *Science in the private interest: Has the lure of profits corrupted biomedcial research?* Lanham, MD: Rowman & Littlefield.

Kroll-Smith, Steve, Phil Brown, and Valerie Gunter. 2000. *Illness and the environment: A reader in contested medicine*. New York: New York University Press.

Kuhn, Thomas. 1962. *The structure of scientific revolutions*. Chicago: University of Chicago Press.

Kulldorff, Martin, Eric J. Feuer, Barry A. Miller, and Laurence S. Freedman. 1997. Breast cancer clusters in the northeast United States: A geographic analysis. *American Journal of Epidemiology* 146: 161–70.

Labreche, France, and Mark Goldberg. 1997. Exposure to organic solvents and breast cancer in women: A hypothesis. *American Journal of Industrial Medicine* 32: 1–14.

Lee, S. Y., M. T. Kim, S. W. Kim, M. S. Song, and S. J. Yoon. 2003. Effect of cohort lifetime lactation on breast cancer risk: A Korean women's cohort study. *International Journal of Cancer* 105: 390–93.

Lerner, Barron. 2001. *The breast cancer wars: Hope, fear, and the pursuit of a cure in twentieth-century America*. New York: Oxford University Press.

Levy, Jonathan, John D. Spengler, Dennis Hlinka, and David Sullivan. 2000. *Estimated public health impacts of criteria pollutant air emissions from the Salem Harbor and Brayton Point power plants*. Cambridge, MA: Harvard School of Public Health.

Lichtenstein, P., N. Holm, P. K. Verkasalo, A. Iliadou, J. Kaprio, M. Koskenvuo, E. Pukkala, A. Skytthe, and K. Hemminki. 2000. Environmental and heritable factors in the causation of cancer—Analyses of cohorts of twins from Sweden, Denmark, and Finland. *New England Journal of Medicine* 343: 78–85.

Lipworth, Loren, L. Renee Bailey, and Dimitrios Trichopoulos. 2000. History of breast-feeding in relation to breast cancer risk: A review of the epidemiologic literature. *Journal of the National Cancer Institute* 92: 302–12.

Lord, Sarah J., Leslie Bernstein, Karen Johnson, Kathi Malone, Linda Weiss, Jill Mc-Donald, and Giske Ursin. 2007. Parity, breastfeeding and breast cancer risk by hormone receptor status in women with late age at first birth—A case control study. Paper presented at the American Association for Cancer Research meeting, Los Angeles.

Lorde, Audre. 1980. *The cancer journals*. San Francisco: Aunt Lute Books.

Love, Susan M., and Karen Lindsey. 1997. The politics of breast cancer. In *Feminist frontiers*, vol. 4, edited by L. Richardson, V. Taylor, and N. Whittier. New York: McGraw-Hill, 384–91.

Malkan, Stacy. 2008. *Not just a pretty face: The ugly side of the beauty industry*. Gabriola Island, BC: New Society Publishers.

Markey, C. M., B. S. Rubin, A. M. Soto, and C. Sonnenschein. 2002. Endocrine disruptors: From wingspread to environmental developmental biology. *Journal of Steroid Biochemistry and Molecular Biology* 83, nos. 1–5: 235–44.

Markowitz, Gerald, and David Rosner. 2002. *Deceit and denial: The deadly politics of industrial pollution*. Berkeley: University of California Press.

Martin, Andrea Ravinett. 2000. Uncovering the truth. *Contra Costa Times* (op-ed).

May, Troy, Susan L. Thomas, and Kathy Robertson. 2001. Breast exam centers hit by overload. *East Bay Business Times*, November 23. http://www.bizjournals.com/eastbay/stories/2001/11/26/story3.html

Mayo Clinic. 2005. *Types of breast cancer*. http://www.mayoclinic.com/health/breast-cancer/HQ00348

McCormick, Sabrina, Phil Brown, and Stephen Zavestoski. 2003. The personal is scientific, the scientific is political: The public paradigm of the environmental breast cancer movement. *Sociological Forum* 18: 545–76.

Meironyté, Daiva, Koidu Norén, and Åke Bergman. 1999. Analysis of polybrominated diphenyl ethers in Swedish human milk: A time-related trend study, 1972–1997. *Journal of Toxicology and Environmental Health* 58: 329–41.

Melbye, Mads, Jan Wohlfahrt, Jørgen H. Olsen, Morten Frisch, Tine Westergaard, Karin Helweg-Larsen, and Per Kragh Andersen. 1997. Induced abortion and the risk of breast cancer. *New England Journal of Medicine* 336: 81–85.

Miller, Anthony B., Teresa To, Cornelia J. Baines, and Claus Wall. 2000. Canadian National Breast Screening Study-2: 13-year results of a randomized trial in women aged 50–59 years. *Journal of the National Cancer Institute* 92: 1490–99.

Milliron, Kara J., and Sofia D. Merajver. 2006. *Breast cancer genetics and clinical practice*. *Michigan Oncology Journal*, Spring 2000.

Mills, Lisa Nicole. 2002. *Science and social context: The regulation of recombinant bovine growth hormone in North America*. McGill-Queen's University Press.

Mills, Paul K., and Richard C. Yang. 2005. Breast cancer risk in Hispanic agricultural workers in California. *International Journal of Occupational and Environmental Health* 11, no. 2: 123–31.

Mintzes, Barbara, Morris L. Barer, Richard L. Kravitz, Arminée Kazanjian, Ken Bassett, Joel Lexchin, Robert G. Evans, Richard Pan, and Stephen A. Marion. 2002. Influence of direct to consumer pharmaceutical advertising and patients' requests on prescribing decisions: Two site cross sectional survey. *British Medical Journal* 324: 278–79.

Mishler, Elliot. 1981. Viewpoint: Critical perspectives on the biomedical model. In *Social contexts of health, illness and patient care*, edited by Elliot Mishler, Lorna Amarasingham, Stuart Hauser, Ramsay Liem, Samel Osherson, and Nancy Waxler. Cambridge: Cambridge University Press, 1–19.

Moffett, J. 2003. Moving beyond the ribbon: An examination of breast cancer advocacy and activism in the US and Canada. *Cultural Dynamics* 15: 287–306.

National Academy of Sciences. 2003. *Increased access to high-quality mammography needed to reduce cancer deaths: Shortage of screening specialists should be addressed to deal with capacity crisis*. Washington, DC: National Academies Press.

National Breast Cancer Awareness Month. 2007. http://www.nbcam.org/about_board _of_sponsors.cfm

National Cancer Institute. 1987. *A guide for developing public education programs on breast cancer*. Bethesda, MD: National Cancer Institute.

———. 2003. *Pregnancy and breast cancer risk*. http://www.cancer.gov/cancer topics/factsheet/Risk/pregnancy

Nelson, Richard R. 1999. The sources of industrial leadership: A perspective on industrial policy. *The Economist* 147, no. 1: 1–18.

New York State Department of Public Health, Surveillance Improvement Initiative 1999. Map 2: Breast Cancer Incidence by zip code, New York State, 1993–1977. Albany: New York State Department of Public Health.http://epi.grants.cancer.gov/ LIBCSP/reports/LIGIS_6_06.html#3

Northern California Cancer Center. 1994. *Greater Bay Area Cancer Registry Report* 5, no. 1.

Occupational Safety and Health Administration. 2005. *Reducing worker exposure to perchloroethylene (PERC) in dry cleaning*. Washington, DC: Occupational Safety and Health Administration. http://www.osha.gov/dsg/guidance/perc.pdf

Oishi, Shinshi. 2002. Effects of butyl paraben on the male reproductive system in mice. *Archives of Toxicology* 76, no. 7: 423–29.

Patandin, S., P. C. Dagnelie, P. G. H. Mulder, E. Op de Coul, J. E. van der Veen, N. Weisglas-Kuperus, and P. J. J. Sauer. 1999. Dietary exposure to polychlorinated biphenyls and dioxins from infancy until adulthood: A comparison between breast-feeding, toddler, and long-term exposure. *Environmental Health Perspectives* 107: 45–51.

Paulsen, Monte. 1993. BCAM scam. *The Nation*. November 15, 557–58.

Pearce, Fant, and Steve Tombs. 1996. Hegemony, risk and governance: "'Social regulation'" and the American chemical industry. *Economy and Society* 25, no. 3: 428–54.

Pedersen, K. L., S. N. Pedersen, L. B. Christiansen, B. Korsgaard, and P. Bjerregaard. 2000. The preservatives ethyl-, propyl-, and butylparaben are oestrogenic in an in vivo fish assay. *Pharmacological Toxicology* 86: 110–13.

Pettigrew, Andrew. 1985. *The awakening giant: Continuity and change in imperial chemical industries*. Hoboken, NJ: Basil Blackwell.

Pisano, Etta D., Michael Schell, Jenny Rollins, C. B. Burns, Beverly Hall, Yuhua Lin, M. Patricia Braeuning, Eithne Burke, and Joseph Holliday. 2000. Has the Mammography Quality Standards Act affected the mammography quality in North Carolina? *American Journal of Roentgenology* 174: 1089–91.

Poliakoff, Martyn, J. Michael Fitzpatrick, Trevor R. Farren, and Paul T. Anastas. 2002. Green chemistry: Science and politics of change. *Science* 297, no. 5582: 807–10.

Polonsky, Michael Jay, and Greg Wood. 2001. Can the overcommercialization of cause-related marketing harm society? *Journal of Macromarketing* 21, no. 1: 8–22.

Public Broadcasting System. 1998. Fooling with nature. Interview conducted with Stephen Safe.

Qaseem, Amir, Vincenza Snow, Katherine Sherif, Mark Aronson, Kevin B. Weiss, and Douglas K. Owens. 2007. Screening mammography for women 40 to 49 years of age: A clinical practice guideline from the American College of Physicians. *Annals of Internal Medicine* 146, no. 7: 511–15.

Rakowski, William, and Melissa A. Clark. 1998. Do groups of women aged 50 to 75 match the national average mammography rate? *American Journal of Preventive Medicine* 15, no. 3: 187–97.

Ramirez, Paulina, and Andrew Tylecote. 2002. *Corporate governance and product innovation: A case study of AstraZeneca.* Sheffield, England: European Commission.

Ransom, Steve. 2006. *Pink ribbons and disinformation: The truth about breast cancer and mammography.* http://www.purewatergazette.net/pinkribbons.htm

Ravdin, P. M., K. A. Cronin, N. Howlander, C. D. Berg, R. T. Chlebowski, E. J. Feuer, B. K. Edwards, and D. A. Berry. The decrease in breast cancer incidence in 2003 in the United States. *New England Journal of Medicine* 356: 1670–74.

Reuters. 2002. PVC cleans up image, but fears EU regulation. May 6.

Ritter, S. K. 2002. Green challenge: Presidential awards recognize innovative synthesis process improvements, and new products that promote pollution prevention. *Chemical Engineering News* 80, no. 26: 26–30. http://www.sourcewatch.org/index.php?title=The_Advancement_of_Sound_Science_Coalition

Robinson, Melissa B. *South Coast Today.* Washington.

Rose, Geoffry. 1992. *The strategy of preventive medicine.* Oxford: Oxford University Press.

Rosenbaum, M. E., and G. M. Roos. 2000. Women's experiences of breast cancer. In *Breast cancer: Society shapes an epidemic,* edited by A. S. Kasper and S. J. Ferguson. New York: Palgrave, 153–82.

Rosser, Sue V. 2000. Controversies in breast cancer research. In *Breast cancer: Society shapes an epidemic,* edited by A. S. Kasper and S. J. Ferguson. New York: Palgrave, 245–70.

Routledge, E. J., J. Parker, J. Odum, J. Ashby, and J. P. Sumpter. 1998. Some alkyl hydroxy benzoate preservatives (parabens) are estrogenic. *Toxicology and Applied Pharmacology* 153: 12–19.

Rudel, Ruthann A., Kathleen R. Attfield, Jessica N. Schifano, and Julia Green Brody. 2007. Chemicals causing mammary gland tumors in animals signal new directions for epidemiology, chemicals testing, and risk assessment for breast cancer prevention. *Cancern* 109, suppl. 12: 2635–66.

Rudel, R. A., D. E. Camann, J. D. Spengler, L. R. Korn, and J. G. Brody. 2003. Phthalates, alkylphenols, pesticides, polybrominated diphenyl ethers, and other endocrine-disrupting compounds in indoor air and dust. *Environmental Science and Technology* 37, no. 20: 4543–53.

Rudel, R. A., P. Geno, G. Sun, A. Yau, J. Spengler, J. Vallarino, and J. G. Brody. 2001. Identification of selected hormonally active agents and animal mammary carcinogens in commercial and residential air and dust samples. *Journal of the Air and Waste Management Association* 51: 499–513.

Ruzek, S. B. 1980. Medical response to women's health activities: Conflict, accommodation and cooptation. *Research in the Sociology of Health Care* 1: 335–54.

Ryerson, B., J. Miller, C. R. Eheman, and M. C. White. 2007. *Use of mammograms among women aged ≥40 years—United States, 2000–2005.* Atlanta: Centers for Disease Control and Prevention, National Center for Chronic Disease Prevention and Health Promotion, Division of Cancer Prevention and Control.

Safe, Stephen. 1997. Xenoestrogens and breast cancer. *New England Journal of Medicine* 337: 1303–4.

Salem News. 2005. *Dust study shows toxins are right under our noses.* March 25. http://www.silentspring.org/news/media-coverage/dust-study-shows-toxins-are -right-under-our-noses

SF Chronicle. 2006. Editorial: Green chemistry for California. *San Francisco Chronicle*, April 3.

Schapiro, Mark. 2005. New power for "Old Europe." *International Journal of Health Services* 35, no. 3: 551–60.

Schneible, C. 2003. http://www.causemarketingforum.com

Senate Environment and Public Works Committee Field Hearing. 2001. Garden City, NY: Adelphi University, June 11.

Sephton, Sandra E., Robert M. Sapolsky, Helena C. Kraemer, and David Spiegel. 2000. Diurnal cortisol rhythm as a predictor of breast cancer survival. *Journal of the National Cancer Institute* 92: 994–1000.

Shamir, R. 2004. The de-radicalization of corporate social responsibility. *Critical Sociology* 30: 669–89.

Shaw, Elizabeth. 2007. Legal toxins in air: GM's truck plant rated among worst polluters, with blessings of EPA. *Flint Journal* First Edition, April 8.

Shills, Judith. 1988. *FDA drug bulletin: A guide for developing public education programs on breast cancer.* Washington, DC: Food and Drug Administration.

Silent Spring Institute. 1998. *The Cape Cod Breast Cancer and Environment Study: Results of the first three years of study.* Newton, MA: Silent Spring Institute.

———. 2006. *Findings of the Cape Cod Breast Cancer and Environment Study.* Newton, MA: Silent Spring Institute.

Smith-Warner, A. Stephanie, Donna Spiegelman, Shiaw-Shyuan Yaun, Piet A. van den Brandt, Aaron R. Folsom, R. Alexandra Goldbohm, Saxon Graham, Lars Holmberg, Geoffrey R. Howe, James R. Marshall, Anthony B. Miller, John D. Potter, Frank E. Speizer, Walter C. Willett, Alicja Wolk, and David J. Hunter. 1998. Alcohol and breast cancer in women: A pooled analysis of cohort studies. *Journal of the American Medical Association* 279: 535–40.

Snedeker, Suzanne M. 2003. Environmental chemicals and breast cancer risk: Where have we been and where are we headed? *Stop the Epidemic: The Newsletter of the Massachusetts Breast Cancer Coalition.* Massachusetts Breast Cancer Coalition. http://mbcc.org/content.php?id=103

Sonnenschein, C., and A. M Soto. 1998. An updated review of environmental estrogen and androgen mimics and antagonists. *Journal of Steroid Biochemistry and Molecular Biology* 65, nos. 1–6: 143–50.

Soto, Ana M., Kerrie L. Chung, and Carlos Sonnenschein. 1994. The pesticides endosulfan, toxaphene, and dieldrin have estrogenic effects on human estrogen-sensitive cells. *Environmental Health Perspectives* 1024: 380–83.

SourceWatch. 2006. The Advancement of Sound Science Coalition. http://www.sourcewatch.org/index.php?title=The_Advancement_of_Sound_Science_Coalition#A_.22Sound_Science.22_Award_for_Gina_Kolata.27s_Reporting_on_Silicon_Breast_Implants

Sporn, M. B. 1996. The war on cancer. *Lancet* 347: 1377–81.

Stabiner, Karen. 1997. *To dance with the devil: The new war on breast cancer; politics, power, people*. New York: Delacorte Press.

Stauber, John C., and Sheldon Rampton. 1995. *Toxic sludge is good for you: Lies, damn lies and the public relations industry*. Monroe, ME: Common Courage Press.

Steingraber, Sandra. 1998. *Living downstream: An ecologist looks at cancer and the environment*. New York: Vintage.

Stellman, S. D., and Q. S. Wang. 1994. Cancer mortality in Chinese immigrants to New York City: Comparison with Chinese in Tianjin and with United States-born whites. *Cancer* 73, no. 4: 1270–75.

Taylor, Graham D., and Patricia E. Sudnick. 1984. *Du Pont and the international chemical industry*. Florence, KY: Gale/Cengage Learning.

Tesh, Sylvia. 1988. *Hidden arguments: Political ideology and disease prevention policy.* New Brunswick, NJ: Rutgers University Press.

Thomas, J. K., B. Qin, D. A. Howell, and B. E. Richardson. 2001. Environmental hazards and rates of female breast cancer mortality in Texas. *Sociological Spectrum* 21, no. 3: 359–75.

Thornton, Joe, and Jack Weinberg. 1993. *Transition planning for the chlorine phaseout: Economic benefits, costs, and opportunities*. Washington, DC: Greenpeace.

Tundo, Pietro, Paul Anastas, David St.C. Black, Joseph Breen, Terrence Collins, Sofia Memoli, Junshi Miyamoto, Martyn Polyakoff, and William Tumas. 2000. Synthetic pathways and processes in green chemistry: Introductory overview. *Pure Applied Chemistry* 72, no. 7: 1207–28.

Vogel, David. 2003. The hare and the tortoise revisited: The new politics of consumer and environmental regulation in Europe. *British Journal of Political Science* 33: 557–80.

Wakefield, J. 2002. New centers to focus on autism and other developmental disorders. *Environmental Health Perspectives* 110: A20–A21.

Warren, Barbour, and Carol Devine. 2004. *Fact sheet #49: Understanding breast cancer risk and risk factors associated with diet and lifestyle*. Ithaca, NY: Program on Breast Cancer and Environmental Risk Factors.

Weisman, Carol S. 1998. *Women's health care: Activist traditions and institutional change*. Baltimore: Johns Hopkins University Press.

———. 2000. Breast cancer policymaking. In *Breast cancer: Society shapes an epidemic*, edited by A. S. Kasper and S. J. Ferguson. New York: Palgrave, 213–44.

Wolff, Mary S., Paolo G. Toniolo, Eric W. Lee, Marilyn Rivera, and Neil Dubin. 1993. Blood levels of organochlorine residues and risk of breast cancer. *Journal of the National Cancer Institute* 85: 648–52.

Wooster, R., S. L. Neuhausen, J. Mangion, Y. Quirk, D. Ford, N. Collins, K. Nguyen, S. Seal, T. Tran, D. Averill, et al. 1994. Localization of a breast cancer susceptibility gene, BRCA2, to chromosome 13q 12–13. *Science* 265, no. 5181: 2088–90.

World Health Organization. 2003. *Global cancer rates could increase by 50% to 15 million by 2020.* http://www.who.int/mediacentre/news/releases/2003/pr27/en

Yeargin-Allsop, Marshalyn. 2003. Prevalence of autism in a US metropolitan area. *Journal of the American Medical Association* 289: 49–55.

Zahm, S. H., and M. H. Ward. 1998. Pesticides and childhood cancer. *Environmental Health Perspectives* 106, suppl. 3: 893–908.

Zones, J. S. 2000. Profits from pain: The political economy of breast cancer. In *Breast cancer: Society shapes an epidemic*, edited by A. S. Kasper and S. J. Ferguson. New York: Palgrave, 119–52.

Index

About the Author

Sabrina McCormick is a Robert Wood Johnson Health and Society scholar at the University of Pennsylvania and was previously assistant professor of environmental science and sociology at Michigan State University. She is the director and producer of the independent feature-length documentary *No Family History*. www.nofamilyhistory.org